Editors

ASIF M. ILYAS
SAQIB REHMAN
GILES R. SCUDERI
FELASFA M. WODAJO

ORTHOPEDIC CLINICS
OF NORTH AMERICA

www.orthopedic.theclinics.com

July 2015 • Volume 46 • Number 3

ELSEVIER

1600 John F. Kennedy Boulevard • Suite 1800 • Philadelphia, Pennsylvania, 19103-2899.

http://www.orthopedic.theclinics.com

ORTHOPEDIC CLINICS OF NORTH AMERICA Volume 46, Number 3
July 2015 ISSN 0030-5898, ISBN-13: 978-0-323-39109-2

Editor: Jennifer Flynn-Briggs
Developmental Editor: Stephanie Wissler

Orthopedic Clinics of North America (ISSN 0030-5898) is published quarterly by Elsevier Inc., 360 Park Avenue South, New York, NY 10010-1710. Months of issue are January, April, July, and October. Business and Editorial Offices: 1600 John F. Kennedy Blvd., Suite 1800, Philadelphia, PA 19103-2899. Customer Service Office: 3251 Riverport Lane, Maryland Heights, MO 63043. Periodicals postage paid at New York, NY and additional mailing offices. Subscription prices are $310.00 per year for (US individuals), $596.00 per year for (US institutions), $365.00 per year (Canadian individuals), $727.00 per year (Canadian institutions), $450.00 per year (international individuals), $727.00 per year (international institutions), $150.00 per year (US students), $220.00 per year (Canadian and international students). Foreign air speed delivery is included in all *Clinics* subscription prices. All prices are subject to change without notice. **POSTMASTER:** Send change of address to *Orthopedic Clinics of North America*, **Elsevier Health Sciences Division, Subscription Customer Service, 3251 Riverport Lane, Maryland Heights, MO 63043. Customer Service (orders, claims, online, change of address): Elsevier Health Sciences Division, Subscription Customer Service, 3251 Riverport Lane, Maryland Heights, MO 63043. Tel: 1-800-654-2452 (U.S. and Canada); 314-447-8871 (outside U.S. and Canada). Fax: 314-447-8029. E-mail:** journalscustomerservice-usa@elsevier. com **(for print support);** journalsonlinesupport-usa@elsevier.com **(for online support).**

Reprints. For copies of 100 or more, of articles in this publication, please contact the Commercial Reprints Department, Elsevier Inc., 360 Park Avenue South, New York, NY 10010-1710. Tel.: 212-633-3874; Fax: 212-633-3820; E-mail: reprints@elsevier. com.

Orthopedic Clinics of North America is covered in *MEDLINE/PubMed (Index Medicus), Cinahl, Excerpta Medica,* and *Cumulative Index to Nursing and Allied Health Literature.*

PROGRAM OBJECTIVE

Orthopedic Clinics of North America offers clinical review articles on the most cutting-edge technologies and techniques in the field, including adult reconstruction, the upper extremity, pediatrics, trauma, oncology, and sports medicine.

TARGET AUDIENCE

Practicing orthopedic surgeons, orthopedic residents, and other healthcare professionals who specialize in orthopedic technologies and techniques for adult reconstruction, the upper extremity, pediatrics, trauma, oncology, and sports medicine.

LEARNING OBJECTIVES

Upon completion of this activity, participants will be able to:
1. Review the risks and outcomes associated with total hip arthroplasty.
2. Recognize methods of pain management in hand surgery.
3. Discuss imaging and treatment of orthopaedic cancers.

ACCREDITATION

The Elsevier Office of Continuing Medical Education (EOCME) is accredited by the Accreditation Council for Continuing Medical Education (ACCME) to provide continuing medical education for physicians.

The EOCME designates this enduring material for a maximum of 15 *AMA PRA Category 1 Credit*(s)™. Physicians should claim only the credit commensurate with the extent of their participation in the activity.

All other health care professionals requesting continuing education credit for this enduring material will be issued a certificate of participation.

DISCLOSURE OF CONFLICTS OF INTEREST

The EOCME assesses conflict of interest with its instructors, faculty, planners, and other individuals who are in a position to control the content of CME activities. All relevant conflicts of interest that are identified are thoroughly vetted by EOCME for fair balance, scientific objectivity, and patient care recommendations. EOCME is committed to providing its learners with CME activities that promote improvements or quality in healthcare and not a specific proprietary business or a commercial interest.

The planning committee, staff, authors and editors listed below have identified no financial relationships or relationships to products or devices they or their spouse/life partner have with commercial interest related to the content of this CME activity:

Daniel C. Acevedo, MD; Stephen Becher, MD; Ajit J. Deshmukh, MD; Neil T. Dion, MD; Jennifer Flynn-Briggs; Anjali Fortna; Viktor J. Hansen, MD; Asif M. Ilyas, MD; Edward W. Jernigan, MD; Constantinos Ketonis, MD, PhD; Joseph F. Konopka, MD, MSc; Frank A. Liporace, MD; Christopher M. Melnic, MD; Daisuke Mori, MD; Shervin Oskouei, MD; Wayne G. Paprosky, MD; Parthiv A. Rathod, MD; Santha Priya; Joshua C. Rozell, MD; Harry E. Rubash, MD; Neil. P. Sheth, MD; Brett Shore, MD; Megan Suermann; Felasfa M. Wodajo, MD; Richard S. Yoon, MD.

The planning committee, staff, authors and editors listed below have identified financial relationships or relationships to products or devices they or their spouse/life partner have with commercial interest related to the content of this CME activity:

Joseph A. Abboud, MD is on the speakers bureau for Integra LifeSciences Corporation; Tornier, Inc.; and DePuy Synthes, is a consultant/advisor for Integra LifeSciences Corporation and Tornier, Inc., and receives royalties/patents from Integra LifeSciences Corporation.

Charles Bragdon, PhD has research support from Zimmer Inc; MAKO Surgical Corp; Biomet, Inc; and DePuy Synthes, and receives royalties/patents from Zimmer Inc.

Fred D. Cushner, MD is on the speakers bureau for ConvaTec, Inc.; Pacira Pharmaceuticals; and Smith & Nephew, has research support from Pacira Pharmaceuticals, and receives royalties/patents from Smith & Nephew.

Kenneth A. Egol, MD is a consultant/advisor for Exactech, Inc, and receives royalties/patents from Lippinocott; Slack Technologies, Inc.; and Exactech, Inc.

Robert J. Esther, MD, MSc is a consultant/advisor for the Musculoskeletal Transplant Foundation.

Andrew A. Freiberg, MD is a consultant/advisor for Zimmer, Inc. and Medtronic, receives royalties/patents from Biomet, Inc. and Zimmer Inc, and has stock ownership in Orthopedic Technology Group and ArthroSurface.

Frederic Liss, MD has research support from Pacira Pharmaceuticals.

Raffy Mirzayan, MD has research support from Arthrex, Inc.; JRF Ortho; and BioD, LLC, receives royalties/patents from Lippincott and Thieme Medical Publishers, Inc., and has stock ownership in Alignmed and Cayenne medical.

Orhun Muratoglu, PhD receives royalties/patents from Zimmer, Inc.; Biomet, Inc.; Corin; ConforMIS; Renovis Surgical Technologies, Inc.; Stryker; Arthrex, Inc.; and Cambridge Polymer Group, Inc., and has stock ownership in Cambridge Polymer Group, Inc.

Surena Namdari, MD, MSc is a consultant/advisor for Bulletproof Bone Designs LLC and Miami Device Solutions, LLC, receives royalties/patents from Elsevier and Miami Device Solutions, LLC, and has research support from DePuy Synthes; Integra LifeSciences Corporation; Tornier, Inc.; and Zimmer Inc.

Saqib Rehman, MD is a consultant/advisor for DePuy Synthes, and receives royalties/patents from Jaypee Brothers Medical

Publishers (P) Ltd.

Giles R. Scuderi, MD, FACS. is on the speakers bureau for ConvaTec, Inc.; Medtronic; and Zimmer Inc, is a consultant/ advisor for Medtronic; Pacira Pharmaceuticals, Inc.; and Zimmer Inc; has research support from Pacira Pharmaceuticals, and receives royalties/patents from Zimmer Inc.

Gerald R. Williams, MD has research support from and receives royalties and patents from DePuy Synthes.

UNAPPROVED/OFF-LABEL USE DISCLOSURE

The EOCME requires CME faculty to disclose to the participants:

1. When products or procedures being discussed are off-label, unlabelled, experimental, and/or investigational (not US Food and Drug Administration [FDA] approved); and

2. Any limitations on the information presented, such as data that are preliminary or that represent ongoing research, interim analyses, and/or unsupported opinions. Faculty may discuss information about pharmaceutical agents that is outside of FDA-approved labelling. This information is intended solely for CME and is not intended to promote off-label use of these medications. If you have any questions, contact the medical affairs department of the manufacturer for the most recent prescribing information.

TO ENROLL

To enroll in the *Orthopedic Clinics of North America* Continuing Medical Education program, call customer service at 1-800-654-2452 or sign up online at http://www.theclinics.com/home/cme. The CME program is available to subscribers for an additional annual fee of USD 215.

METHOD OF PARTICIPATION

In order to claim credit, participants must complete the following:

1. Complete enrolment as indicated above.
2. Read the activity.
3. Complete the CME Test and Evaluation. Participants must achieve a score of 70% on the test. All CME Tests and Evaluations must be completed online.

CME INQUIRIES/SPECIAL NEEDS

For all CME inquiries or special needs, please contact elsevierCME@elsevier.com.

Contributors

EDITORS

ASIF M. ILYAS, MD – *Upper Extremity*
Program Director of Hand Surgery
Fellowship, Rothman Institute; Associate
Professor of Orthopaedic Surgery
Jefferson Medical College, Philadelphia,
Pennsylvania

SAQIB REHMAN, MD – *Trauma*
Director of Orthopaedic Trauma,
Associate Professor of Orthopaedic
Surgery and Sports Medicine, School of
Medicine, Temple University Hospital,
Temple University, Philadelphia,
Pennsylvania

GILES R. SCUDERI, MD – *Adult
Reconstruction*
Vice President, Orthopedic Service Line,
Northshore Long Island Jewish Health
System; Fellowship Director, Adult Knee
Reconstruction Lenox Hill Hospital,
New York, New York

FELASFA M. WODAJO, MD – *Oncology*
Musculoskeletal Tumor Surgery, Medical
Director, Musculoskeletal Oncology, Virginia
Hospital Center; Assistant Professor,
Orthopedic Surgery, Georgetown University
Hospital; Assistant Professor, Orthopedic
Surgery, Virginia Commonwealth University
School of Medicine, Inova Campus, Arlington,
Virginia

AUTHORS

JOSEPH A. ABBOUD, MD
Research Director; Associate Professor,
Shoulder and Elbow Division, The Rothman
Institute, Philadelphia, Pennsylvania

DANIEL C. ACEVEDO, MD
Department of Orthopedic Surgery, Kaiser
Permanente, Baldwin Park, Panorama City,
California

STEPHEN BECHER, MD
Musculoskeletal Oncology Fellow, Emory
University, Atlanta, Georgia

CHARLES BRAGDON, PhD
Massachusetts General Hospital, Boston,
Massachusetts

FRED D. CUSHNER, MD
Assistant Professor, Hofstra North
Shore-Long Island Jewish School of Medicine;
Chief of Orthopedics, Southside Hospital,
New York, New York

AJIT J. DESHMUKH, MD
Assistant Professor, NYU Hospital for Joint
Diseases/NYU Langone Medical Center,
VA New York Harbor Healthcare system,
New York, New York

NEIL T. DION, MD
Department of Orthopaedic Surgery,
Massachusetts General Hospital, Boston,
Massachusetts

KENNETH A. EGOL, MD
Vice Chairman of Education, Professor,
Program Director, Division of Orthopaedic
Trauma, Department of Orthopaedic Surgery/
NYU Hospital for Joint Diseases, NYU Langone
Medical Center, New York, New York

ROBERT J. ESTHER, MD, MSc
Associate Professor and Residency Program
Director, Department of Orthopaedics,
University of North Carolina, Chapel Hill,
North Carolina

ANDREW A. FREIBERG, MD
Arthroplasty Service Chief and Vice Chair,
Department of Orthopedic Surgery, Yawkey
Center, Massachusetts General Hospital,
Boston, Massachusetts

VIKTOR J. HANSEN, MD
Harris Orthopedic Laboratory, Department of
Orthopedics, Massachusetts General Hospital,
Boston, Massachusetts

ASIF M. ILYAS, MD
Program Director of Hand Surgery
Fellowship, Rothman Institute; Associate
Professor of Orthopaedic Surgery
Jefferson Medical College, Philadelphia,
Pennsylvania

EDWARD W. JERNIGAN, MD
Department of Orthopaedics, University of
North Carolina School of Medicine, University
of North Carolina, Chapel Hill, North Carolina

CONSTANTINOS KETONIS, MD, PhD
Resident, Rothman Institute and Department of
Tissue Engineering and Regenerative
Medicine, Thomas Jefferson University,
Philadelphia, Pennsylvania

JOSEPH F. KONOPKA, MD, MSc
Adult Reconstructive Service, Department of
Orthopedics, Massachusetts General
Hospital, Boston, Massachusetts

FRANK A. LIPORACE, MD
Director, Orthopaedic Trauma Research;
Associate Professor, Division of Orthopaedic
Trauma, Department of Orthopaedic Surgery,
NYU Hospital for Joint Diseases, New York,
New York

FREDERIC LISS, MD
Rothman Institute, Thomas Jefferson
University, Philadelphia, Pennsylvania

CHRISTOPHER M. MELNIC, MD
Orthopaedic Resident, Department of
Orthopaedic Surgery, University of
Pennsylvania, Philadelphia,
Pennsylvania

RAFFY MIRZAYAN, MD
Co-Director of Sports Medicine;
Director of Cartilage Restoration; Director
of Orthopaedic Resident Education,
Kaiser Permanente; Clinical Professor,
Department of Orthopaedic Surgery, University
of Southern California Keck School of
Medicine, Baldwin Park, California

DAISUKE MORI, MD
Kyoto Shimogamo Hospital, Kyoto,
Japan

ORHUN MURATOGLU, PhD
Massachusetts General Hospital, Boston,
Massachusetts

SURENA NAMDARI, MD, MSc
The Rothman Institute, Philadelphia,
Pennsylvania

SHERVIN OSKOUEI, MD
Assistant Professor, Department of
Orthopaedic Surgery, Emory University,
Atlanta, Georgia

WAYNE G. PAPROSKY, MD
Professor of Orthopaedic Surgery, Midwest
Orthopaedics, Rush University, Chicago,
Illinois

PARTHIV A. RATHOD, MD
Clinical Instructor, NYU Hospital for
Joint Diseases/NYU Langone Medical
Center; Chief of Orthopedics,
Woodhull Hospital, New York,
New York

JOSHUA C. ROZELL, MD
Orthopaedic Resident, Department of
Orthopaedic Surgery, University of
Pennsylvania, Philadelphia,
Pennsylvania

HARRY E. RUBASH, MD
Chief of Orthopedic Surgery,
Department of Orthopedic Surgery,
Yawkey Center, Massachusetts General
Hospital, Boston, Massachusetts

NEIL P. SHETH, MD
Assistant Professor of Orthopaedic Surgery,
Department of Orthopaedic Surgery, University
of Pennsylvania, Philadelphia, Pennsylvania

BRETT SHORE, MD
Department of Orthopedic Surgery, Kaiser
Permanente, Baldwin Park, Panorama City,
California

GERALD R. WILLIAMS, MD
The Rothman Institute, Philadelphia,
Pennsylvania

RICHARD S. YOON, MD
Resident, Division of Orthopaedic Trauma,
Department of Orthopaedic Surgery, NYU
Hospital for Joint Diseases, New York,
New York

NEIL P. SHETH, MD
Assistant Professor of Orthopaedic Surgery,
Department of Orthopaedic Surgery, University
of Pennsylvania, Philadelphia, Pennsylvania

BRETT SHORE, MD
Department of Orthopedic Surgery, Kaiser
Permanente, Baldwin Park, Panorama City,
California

GERALD R. WILLIAMS, MD
The Rothman Institute, Philadelphia,
Pennsylvania

RICHARD S. YOON, MD
Resident, Division of Orthopaedic Trauma,
Department of Orthopaedic Surgery, NYU
Hospital for Joint Diseases, New York,
New York

Contents

Adult Reconstruction

Preface   xiii

Giles R. Scuderi

**Durability of Highly Cross-Linked Polyethylene in Total Hip and Total
Knee Arthroplasty**   321

Neil T. Dion, Charles Bragdon, Orhun Muratoglu, and Andrew A. Freiberg

> This article reviews the history of the development of highly cross-linked polyeth-
> ylene (HXLPE) and provides an in-depth review of the clinical results regarding the
> durability of HXLPE used in total hip arthroplasty (THA) and total knee arthroplasty
> (TKA). The use of polyethylene as a bearing surface has contributed to the success
> of THA and TKA; however, polyethylene wear and osteolysis can lead to failure.
> Ongoing clinical and retrieval studies are required to analyze outcomes at longer-
> term follow-up.

Management of Severe Femoral Bone Loss in Revision Total Hip Arthroplasty   329

Neil P. Sheth, Christopher M. Melnic, Joshua C. Rozell, and Wayne G. Paprosky

> Femoral bone loss is a complex problem in revision total hip arthroplasty. The Paprosky
> classification is used when determining the degree and location of bone loss. Meticu-
> lous operative planning is essential where severe bone loss is a concern. One must
> correctly identify the bone loss pattern, safely remove the existing components, and
> proceed with the proper reconstruction technique based on the pattern of bone
> loss. This article discusses the etiology and classification of bone loss, clinical and
> radiographic evaluation, components of effective preoperative planning, and clinical
> results of various treatment options with a focus on more severe bone loss patterns.

**Reducing Blood Loss in Bilateral Total Knee Arthroplasty with Patient-Specific
Instrumentation**   343

Parthiv A. Rathod, Ajit J. Deshmukh, and Fred D. Cushner

> Patient-specific instrumentation (PSI) in total knee arthroplasty (TKA) has been intro-
> duced to obtain consistent alignment, prevent instrumentation of the medullary ca-
> nal and improve operating room efficiency. This article compares simultaneous
> bilateral TKA performed with and without the use of PSI in terms of surgical time;
> blood loss and transfusion requirements; length-of-stay; early thromboembolic
> events; and complication rates. There was a trend to reduced total blood loss (as
> measured by drop in hemoglobin values) and lower transfusion rate after surgery.
> Further research in the form of high quality randomized trials and cost-benefit ana-
> lyses may help in further consolidation of these findings.

**Risk Assessment Tools Used to Predict Outcomes of Total Hip and Total Knee
Arthroplasty**   351

Joseph F. Konopka, Viktor J. Hansen, Harry E. Rubash, and Andrew A. Freiberg

> This article reviews recently proposed clinical tools for predicting risks and out-
> comes in total hip arthroplasty and total knee arthroplasty patients. Additionally,

we share the Massachusetts General Hospital experience with using the Risk Assessment and Prediction Tool to predict the need for an extended care facility after total joint arthroplasty.

Trauma

Preface   xv

Saqib Rehman

Definitive Fixation of Tibial Plateau Fractures   363

Richard S. Yoon, Frank A. Liporace, and Kenneth A. Egol

Tibial plateau fractures present in a wide spectrum of injury severity and pattern, each requiring a different approach and strategy to achieve good clinical outcomes. Achieving those outcomes starts with a thorough evaluation and preoperative planning period, which leads to choosing the most appropriate surgical approach and fixation strategy. Through a case-based approach, this article presents the necessary pearls, techniques, and strategies to maximize outcomes and minimize complications for some of the more commonly presenting plateau fracture patterns.

Upper Extremity

Preface   xvii

Asif M. Ilyas

Orthopedic Applications of Acellular Human Dermal Allograft for Shoulder and Elbow Surgery   377

Daniel C. Acevedo, Brett Shore, and Raffy Mirzayan

Shoulder and elbow tendon injuries are some of the most challenging problems to treat surgically. Tendon repairs in the upper extremity can be complicated by poor tendon quality and, often times, poor healing. Extracellular matrices, such as human dermal allografts, have been used to augment tendon repairs in shoulder and elbow surgery. The indications and surgical techniques regarding the use of human dermal allograft continue to evolve. This article reviews the basic science, rationale for use, and surgical applications of human dermal allograft in shoulder and elbow tendon injuries.

Glenoid Bone Loss in Anatomic Shoulder Arthroplasty: Literature Review and Surgical Technique   389

Daisuke Mori, Joseph A. Abboud, Surena Namdari, and Gerald R. Williams

Despite major advances in total shoulder arthroplasty, management of severe posterior glenoid bone loss remains controversial. Several companies have provided alternative treatment options for type C glenoids associated with posterior subluxation of the humeral head. However, preoperative planning, proper selection of glenoid size, and recognition of the operative pitfalls are crucial for successful outcomes. This article presents a review of the literature and the surgical technique for management of severe posterior glenoid bone loss.

Pain Management Strategies in Hand Surgery   399

Constantinos Ketonis, Asif M. Ilyas, and Frederic Liss

Modern anesthetic agents have allowed for the rapid expansion of ambulatory surgery, particularly in hand surgery. The choice between general anesthesia, peripheral regional blocks, regional intravenous anesthesia (Bier block), local block with sedation, and the recently popularized wide-awake hand surgery depends on several variables, including the type and duration of the procedure and patient characteristics, coexisting conditions, location, and expected length of the procedure. This article discusses the various perioperative and postoperative analgesic options to optimize the hand surgical patient's experience.

Oncology

Preface   xix

Felasfa M. Wodajo

PET Imaging in Sarcoma   409

Stephen Becher and Shervin Oskouei

PET imaging has been evaluated in five areas of sarcoma diagnosis and treatment: biopsy guidance, therapeutic monitoring, tumor detection and grading, tumor staging, and prognostication. Current evidence does not include any cost-benefit analysis showing a decreased number of invasive procedures from false-positive results. There is overlap from more conventional imaging and PET imaging without obvious added benefit from information gained from PET/computed tomography scanning. Use as a routine test in patients with sarcoma cannot be recommended. Use in specific histologic subtypes with differing patterns of metastasis or in monitoring those cases undergoing neoadjuvant chemotherapy needs further study before PET/computed tomography becomes standard of care for patients with sarcoma.

Soft Tissue Masses for the General Orthopedic Surgeon   417

Edward W. Jernigan and Robert J. Esther

Soft tissue sarcomas are a rare, heterogeneous group of malignancies that should be included in the differential diagnosis for any patient presenting with a soft tissue mass. This article reviews strategies for differentiating between benign and malignant soft tissue masses. Epidemiology, appropriate workup, and treatment of soft tissue sarcomas are reviewed.

Index   429

ORTHOPEDIC CLINICS OF NORTH AMERICA

FORTHCOMING ISSUES

Beginning with the July 2013 issue, *Orthopedic Clinics of North America* began to appear in this new format. Rather than focusing on a single topic, each issue contains articles on key areas in orthopedics—adult reconstruction, upper extremity, trauma, pediatrics and oncology. Articles on sports medicine and foot and ankle will also be included on a regular basis. As the practice of orthopedics has become more specialized, the format of one topic per issue is no longer fulfilling our readers' needs. The new format is intended to address these changing needs.

Orthopedic Clinics of North America continues to publish a print issue four times a year, in January, April, July, and October. Articles from our print issues are available on http://www.orthopedic.theclinics.com/.

THE CLINICS ARE AVAILABLE ONLINE!
Access your subscription at:
www.theclinics.com

Adult Reconstruction

Preface

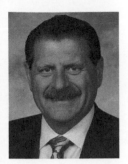

Giles R. Scuderi, MD
Editor

There have been tremendous improvements in total joint arthroplasty over the past few decades, and the demand for total hip and total knee arthroplasty continues to grow. In this issue of *Orthopedic Clinics of North America*, we cover several current topics in total joint arthroplasty that have relevance to contemporary practices.

The first article is by Dion and colleagues on the durability of highly cross-linked polyethylene in total hip and total knee arthroplasty. Here, the authors review the development of highly cross-linked polyethylene and provide an in-depth review of the clinical results, which reveal improved in vivo wear characteristics and decreased osteolysis from short-term to 10-year follow-up. Ongoing long-term clinical studies and registry data will further define the ultimate benefits of highly cross-linked polyethylene.

Inherent to the increased utilization of total hip arthroplasty is an associated burden of revision surgical procedures. In the article by Sheth and colleagues on management of severe femoral bone loss in revision total hip arthroplasty, the authors review the cause of femoral bone loss, associated classification systems, clinical and radiographic patient evaluation, components of effective preoperative planning, and clinical results of various treatment options.

Deceased blood loss in total knee arthroplasty can impact the clinical outcome. In the article by Rathod and colleagues, the authors describe their experience with reducing blood loss in bilateral total knee arthroplasty utilizing patient-specific instrumentation. Avoidance of intramedullary instrumentation with patient-specific guides appears to result in reduced blood loss, reduced transfusion requirement, as well as a decreased risk of systemic embolization. Performed by a high-volume knee surgeon, these results may not be applicable to lower-volume and less-experienced surgeons performing simultaneous bilateral total knee arthroplasty.

As the incidence of total hip and total knee arthroplasty continues to rise, so do patient expectations. A variety of clinical tools have been developed over the last decade to predict a variety of outcomes in total joint arthroplasty patients. Konopka and coauthors review the risk assessment tools used to predict outcomes of total hip and total knee arthroplasty. Such tools may aid efficient care delivery as demand for total joint arthroplasty increases.

Giles R. Scuderi, MD
210 East 64th Street
New York, NY 10065, USA

E-mail address:
gscuderi@nshs.edu

Orthop Clin N Am 46 (2015) xiii
http://dx.doi.org/10.1016/j.ocl.2015.03.005
0030-5898/15/$ – see front matter © 2015 Published by Elsevier Inc.

orthopedic.theclinics.com

Durability of Highly Cross-Linked Polyethylene in Total Hip and Total Knee Arthroplasty

Neil T. Dion, MD*, Charles Bragdon, PhD, Orhun Muratoglu, PhD, Andrew A. Freiberg, MD

KEYWORDS

- Highly cross-linked polyethylene • Total hip arthroplasty • Total knee arthroplasty • Osteolysis
- Vitamin E

KEY POINTS

- The durability of modern highly cross-linked polyethylene in total hip arthroplasty and total knee arthroplasty has been excellent.
- The manufacturing process leads to free radical generation, which leads to oxidation and reduced mechanical properties.
- Postprocessing modifications such as remelting and vitamin E doping reduce the risk of oxidation.
- Ten-year wear and survival data for highly cross-linked polyethylene continue to be favorable, but the long-term durability has not yet been demonstrated in vivo.

INTRODUCTION

Total hip arthroplasty (THA) and total knee arthroplasty (TKA) have excellent track records with regards to pain relief and improvement of function. Over the past several decades, there have been significant improvements in the engineering and materials science of bearing surfaces. The use of highly cross-linked polyethylene (HXLPE) in large-joint arthroplasty has led to improved outcomes, particularly for THA. This article briefly reviews the history of the development of HXLPE and provides an in-depth review of the clinical results regarding the durability of HXLPE in THA and TKA.

Sir John Charnley attempted to develop a low-friction arthroplasty with the use of Teflon-bearing surfaces.[1] The wear characteristics of this material were unsatisfactory with dramatic early failure from wear. He eventually transitioned to metal-on-polyethylene THA. Charnley's recognition that polyethylene was a good bearing surface revolutionized hip arthroplasty.

The use of polyethylene as a bearing surface contributed to the success of THA and TKA; however, it was not without complications. Ultra-high-molecular-weight polyethylene (UHMWPE) wear can lead to a local reaction that results in bone resorption or osteolysis.[2] **Fig. 1** demonstrates a

Disclosures: Charles Bragdon, PhD receives research support and royalties from Zimmer; Orhun Muratoglu, PhD receives research support from Depuy/Synthes, Biomet, Zimmer, and Stryker. He receives royalties from Biomet, Zimmer, Corin, Conformis, Alchimist, Aston Medical, Ceramtech, Maxx Orthopedics, Iconacy, Renovis, Arthrex, Stryker, Orthopedic Technology Group, and Cambridge Polymer Group; Andrew Freiberg, MD is a consultant for Zimmer, Medtronic and CeramTec. He receives royalties from Zimmer and Biomet. He has ownership in ArthroSurface.
Department of Orthopaedic Surgery, Massachusetts General Hospital, 55 Fruit Street, Suite 3700, Boston, MA 02114, USA
* Corresponding author.
E-mail address: NDion1@Partners.org

Orthop Clin N Am 46 (2015) 321–327
http://dx.doi.org/10.1016/j.ocl.2015.02.001
0030-5898/15/$ – see front matter © 2015 Elsevier Inc. All rights reserved.

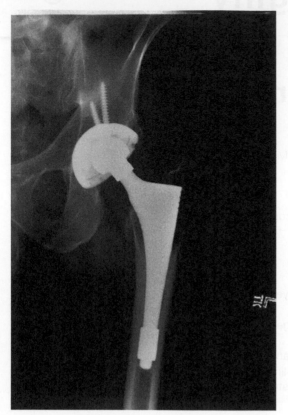

Fig. 1. A radiograph of a patient with osteolysis around the acetabular and femoral components due to polyethylene wear following THA.

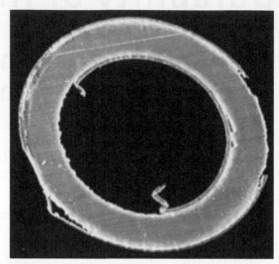

Fig. 2. A thin section of a retrieved conventional polyethylene insert demonstrating white banding due to subsurface oxidation of the material.

radiograph of a patient with osteolysis around the acetabular and femoral components due to polyethylene wear following THA. Polyethylene wear and osteolysis have been an important cause of long-term failure of THA. The technique of highly cross-linking polyethylene was developed to make the material more resistant to wear and reduce the incidence of this mechanism of failure in arthroplasty.

Ionizing γradiation is used to highly cross-link polyethylene by breaking hydrogen-carbon bonds, which then allows molecular cross-linking, thus improving the wear characteristics of the polymer but leading to the creation of free radicals. These free radicals can allow the polyethylene to oxidize over time and decrease the material's fracture resistance. Irradiation with oxygen present potentiates this detrimental effect and leads to early oxidation.[3] Fig. 2 demonstrates a thin section of a retrieved conventional polyethylene insert demonstrating white banding due to subsurface oxidation of the material. The result of oxidation is a reduction in the mechanical properties leading to a more brittle polyethylene. Delamination of the polyethylene in TKA can be seen under these

circumstances. Cracking can compromise the locking mechanism. As a result, modern components are sterilized and irradiated in oxygen-free environments with the use of inert gas or gas sterilization.

Postradiation processing techniques have been developed to reduce or eliminate the number of free radicals that remain after γ irradiation. Remelting, annealing, and mechanical elimination of free radicals are 3 well-described techniques that have been used to improve the oxidative stability of HXLPE. When remelting, the polyethylene is heated past its melting point to eliminate crystals and allow the remaining free radicals to cross-link with each other. Remelting creates a material with no free radicals but slightly decreases mechanical strength and fracture toughness. During annealing, the maximum temperature is less than the melting point. Annealing results in a greater number of remaining free radicals compared with melting but may be less detrimental to the mechanical properties and J-fracture toughness.[4]

A more recent technique for reducing oxidation in polyethylene involves manufacturing the polymer to include an antioxidant. The antioxidants can stabilize free radicals that exist as a byproduct of manufacturing and protect against future in vivo oxidation as well. Vitamin E has been the most commonly used antioxidant for this purpose. Irganox is another antioxidant that was recently introduced for TKA. Laboratory data have suggested that the use of vitamin E in polyethylene can decrease oxidation characteristics without negatively impacting the mechanical qualities. It eliminates the need for melting. There is also some evidence that it is associated with a reduction in the biologic activity of wear particle.[5] Long-term clinical data are not yet available, but clinical studies are ongoing. Greene and colleagues[6] presented a multicenter prospective study of 977 THA patients. The vitamin E–diffused polyethylene group had −0.04 mm/yr head penetration at 5 years and no evidence of osteolysis. An radiostereometric analysis study of vitamin E UHMWPE by the same group demonstrated 0.05-mm median head penetration in 47 patients at 5 years.[7]

The types of wear that most frequently impact implanted polyethylene in THA and TKA are adhesive, abrasive, and third-body wear. Adhesive wear is an expected wear pattern in arthroplasty that is due to the friction between the polyethylene and the metal or ceramic-bearing surface with which it articulates. Abrasive wear occurs because of a harder surface sliding against a softer surface. In this case, polyethylene is the softer surface. **Fig. 3** demonstrates the articular surface of a highly cross-linked and melted polyethylene insert retrieved because of sepsis at 5 years showing retention of the original machine marks, indicating extremely low wear. **Fig. 4** shows a retrieved conventional polyethylene tibial insert demonstrating delamination and pitting due to subsurface oxidation as well as loss of material due to adhesive and abrasive wear. Third-body wear is caused by some substance other than the prosthesis causing abrasion of the polyethylene. This substance is most often a piece of bone, cement, or metal in arthroplasty. HXLPE retrievals can sometimes show surface changes that appear to be wear but are just scratches. The material restores its form because of shape memory.

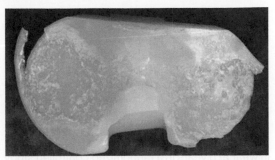

Fig. 4. A retrieved conventional polyethylene tibial insert demonstrating delamination and pitting due to subsurface oxidation as well as loss of material due to adhesive and abrasive wear.

HIGHLY CROSS-LINKED POLYETHYLENE IN TOTAL HIP ARTHROPLASTY

Both biomechanical and clinical studies have shown an advantage to the use of HXLPE over non-cross-linked polyethylene in the hip. In a retrieval study by Muratoglu and colleagues,[8] conventional polyethylene showed more scratching and increased loss of machining marks when compared with HXLPE. Minoda and colleagues[9] reported on wear particle analysis of HXLPE from a failed THA and found that not only were fewer wear particles generated than with conventional UHMWPE but also the particles from HXLPE were smaller and rounder. They hypothesized that this may be associated with a less vigorous macrophage response to wear in HXLPE. Although simulator studies showed marked improvements in wear with HXLPE via adhesive and abrasive wear mechanisms, it should be noted that third-body wear was not significantly improved with the use of HXLPE in a simulator study.[10]

Clinical studies have shown improved wear rates at short-term, mid-term, and now long-term follow-up. Digas and colleagues[11] showed 62% lower proximal penetration with HXLPE over conventional polyethylene at 2 years after surgery using radiostereometry. The HXLPE in that study was compression-molded, γ-irradiated in nitrogen and remelted. Rohrl and colleagues[12] also showed a marked reduction in wear at 2 years with the use of HXLPE that was irradiated in an inert environment and heat annealed with no evidence of any clinical disadvantage. The use of HXLPE with large head arthroplasty also showed excellent wear rates (0.06 mm/yr) at 3 years.[13] Bragdon and colleagues[14] used radiostereometry and found that HXLPE shows acceptable wear rates with large head arthroplasty in ram-extruded, irradiated, and remelted HXLPE used with 36- and 40-mm heads. These results have also been shown to be applicable to younger populations. Ayers and

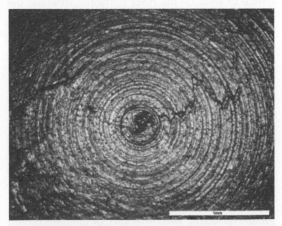

Fig. 3. The articular surface of a highly cross-linked and melted polyethylene insert retrieved due to sepsis at 5 years showing retention of the original machine marks, indicating extremely low wear.

colleagues[15] showed improved wear rates with irradiated and melted HXLPE over conventional UHMWPE in a cohort with mean age of 58.

Dorr and colleagues[16] published 5-year data showing a reduced linear wear rate in ram-extruded electron-beam-irradiated and melted HXLPE with an annual linear wear rate that was only 45% of the rate seen with conventional polyethylene in their radiograph-based clinical study. Engh and colleagues[17] showed a 95% reduction in wear at 5 years in a randomized controlled study comparing γ-irradiated and heat-treated HXLPE with conventional UHMWPE. That study also revealed decreased osteolysis in the HXLPE group compared with the standard UHMWPE group. Multiple other studies have demonstrated an advantage of HXLPE at this time point in both cemented and uncemented components.[18,19]

Meta-analyses and systematic reviews have supported the evidence presented by smaller trials demonstrating that wear rates are reduced with HXLPE over conventional UHMWPE.[20,21] These results have been seen among various manufacturers with differing component designs and locking mechanisms and in many different countries across a variety of hip arthroplasty patient populations.

As expected, the improvements in wear rates have been seen in association with a reduction in osteolysis.[17] A systematic review looking at 9 such studies found an odds ratio of 0.13 for risk of osteolysis in HXLPE compared with conventional UHMWPE.[20] Osteolysis, which was one of the largest challenges facing arthroplasty surgeons, has not been reported at a clinically significant level with the use of HXLPE.

Longer-term data are now becoming available on HXLPE in THA. Bragdon and colleagues[22] published a multicenter study including a cohort with minimum follow-up of 10 years. Again, HXLPE showed wear rates less than the threshold for clinical osteolysis. The authors also found that patient-reported outcomes were comparable with previously published standards for THA.

The data have clearly shown improved wear results with HXLPE over conventional UHMWPE. Manufacturing methods differ for HXLPE, but there are minimal differences in the clinical results for the currently used manufacturing processes of HXLPE up to 10 years out. At longer-term follow-up of 15 and 20 years, the manufacturing differences outlined in the introduction may lead to clinical differences in the device performance. Only time and well-designed outcome studies will provide clinicians, patients, and device manufacturers with this information.

HIGHLY CROSS-LINKED POLYETHYLENE IN TOTAL KNEE ARTHROPLASTY

HXLPE was introduced to TKA later than it was introduced in THA. This later introduction was partially because osteolysis with UHMWPE has not been seen as frequently in TKA as it has been seen in THA; however, it can lead to the need for revision surgery.[23] Although clinically significant osteolysis is less common, delamination and backside wear of polyethylene liners in TKA have been an issue. The slower adaption to TKA was also partly due to concerns over the decreased mechanical properties associated with highly cross-linking and melting the polymer. The forces seen by the polyethylene in TKA are different from those seen by the HXPLE in THA. There was concern that the reduced fatigue strength would be a bigger issue in TKA; this was particularly a concern for posterior-stabilized (PS) implants whereby some had theorized the potential for tibial postfractures.[24] Some companies have modified the manufacturing methods to address these concerns by irradiating their HXLPE for TKA to lower levels than those used for HXLPE in THA. These mechanical concerns have not been supported by clinical literature thus far. There are only 2 reported UHMWPE tibial postfractures that were noted in the authors' literature review, and this study was a case report.[25] None of the larger series have demonstrated a postfracture.

Biomechanical studies were performed using HXLPE inserts in knee simulators. Hermida and colleagues[26] tested sequentially cross-linked and annealed inserts and electron beam–irradiated and remelted inserts against inserts γ-irradiated in air on a simulator of malaligned knee arthroplasty. After one million cycles, the authors noted no evidence of wear on the HXLPE inserts, whereas the inserts that were γ-irradiated in air showed significant damage.[26] Muratoglu and colleagues[27] compared the resistance to delamination of HXLPE with standard UHMWPE in a simulator study after accelerated aging. They found increased wear, oxidation, and delamination in the control group compared with the HXLPE group.[27]

Wang and colleagues[28] tested sequentially irradiated and annealed cruciate-retaining (CR) and PS inserts on a wear simulator against conventional high-molecular-weight polyethylene inserts. They found 68% less wear on CR polyethylene inserts and 64% less wear on PS inserts. They found no significant difference in tensile modulus, yield strength, or ultimate tensile strength between sequentially irradiated and annealed polyethylene and standard UHMWPE. Utzschneider and colleagues[29] also found a reduction in wear with sequentially irradiated and annealed polyethylene compared with standard polyethylene. This result was seen in both fixed and mobile-bearing polyethylene inserts in their study.[29]

Similar to the hip literature, HXLPE in TKA has been shown to generate fewer, rounder, and smaller wear particles when compared with standard UHMWPE,[30] as was shown in an in vivo study using analysis of synovial fluid. These particles may be less biologically stimulating than the particles from conventional UHMWPE.

Given the results seen in biomechanical testing, clinical trials have been performed looking at HXLPE in TKA. Registry data are also available for these inserts. Hodrick and colleagues[31] looked at 100 patients retrospectively at an average follow-up of 75 months and found no subjects with HXLPE had undergone revision. There was no evidence of tibial loosening or polyethylene fracture in their HXLPE group.

Long and colleagues[32] looked at 120 consecutive posterior stabilized TKAs with HXLPE inserts. The polyethylene in their study was irradiated and melted. Mean follow-up time was 52 months. There were 3 revisions in the cohort during the time period, but none of these were related to failure of the HXLPE insert. At the time of revision, none of the liners showed visible signs of wear or failure. There were no progressive radiolucencies on the final radiographic follow-up.

Minoda and colleagues[33] reported on the clinical follow-up of 202 consecutive TKA. They found no differences between conventional UHMWPE and HXLPE at 2-year follow-up in terms of range of motion or Knee Society Score. There were no revisions or evidence of osteolysis in either group.

VITAMIN E STABILIZED HIGHLY CROSS-LINKED POLYETHYLENE

Concerns over the reduced mechanical properties seen in HXLPE associated with remelting or heat annealing led developers to seek alternative methods of stabilization of free radicals. Vitamin E has been used for this purpose with success in vitro, and some of these results are reviewed here. Although biomechanical data are promising, peer-reviewed clinical data for knee applications are not yet available. Multiple studies are currently underway that should help clarify the role of vitamin E stabilized HXLPE.

Wannomae and colleagues[34] performed a biomechanical study to evaluate the wear of vitamin E stabilized polyethylene in unidirectional reciprocating motion. No delamination was seen with induced accelerated aging of the liners. The

same group noted improved wear resistance and fatigue strength in α-tocopherol doped polyethylene compared with standard UHMWPE.[35]

Haider and colleagues[36] used an accelerated aging model to compare α-tocopherol stabilized HXLPE with a remelted HXLPE. They found increased oxidation in the remelted HXLPE. In addition, the vitamin E–stabilized HXLPE had better fatigue crack propagation resistance and better small punch mechanical properties compared with the remelted polyethylene. The reduction in wear was seen in both CR and PS polyethylene liners. Despite the encouraging clinical data and growing frequency of use in arthroplasty, long-term clinical studies regarding the role of vitamin E are needed.

SUMMARY

The existing literature definitively shows that HXLPE has improved laboratory and in vivo wear characteristics and decreased osteolysis from short-term to 10-year follow-up in THA. Biomechanical studies suggest this trend will continue to be seen, but ongoing research is required to analyze clinical outcomes at longer-term follow-up. Current data have shown minimal differences in the clinical results for the currently used manufacturing processes of HXLPE up to 10 years. At longer-term follow-up at 15 and 20 years, the manufacturing differences may lead to performance differences in the data. Only time and ongoing research will definitively provide this information.

The biomechanical data for TKA also suggest reduced wear and reduced delamination with the use of HXLPE compared with conventional UHMWPE. The theorized risks associated with reduced mechanical characteristics of the HXLPE have not been shown to be an issue in the short-term clinical studies that are available. Longer-term follow-up is required to improve the understanding of the clinical benefits and risks of using HXLPE in TKA.

Agents such as vitamin E have been used to stabilize free radicals generated during the manufacturing of HXLPE. In vitro testing of this polyethylene has been very promising, but at this point, clinical studies are not yet available for publication.

There have been tremendous improvements in arthroplasty over the past several decades. The improved manufacturing of HXLPE has contributed to improved outcomes. Long-term clinical studies and registry data will be instrumental in defining and quantifying the relative benefits and risks of the various manufacturing methodologies described for the production of HXLPE for use in TKA and THA.

ACKNOWLEDGMENTS

The authors would like to acknowledge the significant contributions of Ms Ida Lindman for her work in the preparation of this article.

REFERENCES

1. Charnley J. Using Teflon in arthroplasty of the hip-joint. J Bone Joint Surg Am 1966;48:819.
2. Harris WH. Osteolysis and particle disease in hip replacement. A review. Acta Orthop Scand 1994; 65:113–23.
3. Premnath V, Harris WH, Jasty M, et al. Gamma sterilization of UHMWPE articular implants: an analysis of the oxidation problem. Ultra high molecular weight poly ethylene. Biomaterials 1996;17:1741–53.
4. Muratoglu OK, Merrill EW, Bragdon CR, et al. Effect of radiation, heat, and aging on in vitro wear resistance of polyethylene. Clin Orthop Relat Res 2003;(417):253–62.
5. Bladen CL, Teramura S, Russell SL, et al. Analysis of wear, wear particles, and reduced inflammatory potential of vitamin E ultrahigh-molecular-weight polyethylene for use in total joint replacement. J Biomed Mater Res B Appl Biomater 2013;101:458–66.
6. Greene M, Sillesen N, Nebergall A, et al. 5 Year long-term multicenter outcomes with vitamin E polyethylene liners and porous-titanium coated shells. AAHKS 24th Annual Meeting. Dallas (TX), November 8, 2014.
7. Greene M, Nebergall A, Sillesen N, et al. 5 Year RSA evaluation of vitamin E infused polyethylene wear and stability of acetabular femoral components. AAHKS 24th Annual Meeting. Dallas (TX), November 8, 2014.
8. Muratoglu OK, Greenbaum ES, Bragdon CR, et al. Surface analysis of early retrieved acetabular polyethylene liners: a comparison of conventional and highly crosslinked polyethylenes. J Arthroplasty 2004;19:68–77.
9. Minoda Y, Kobayashi A, Sakawa A, et al. Wear particle analysis of highly crosslinked polyethylene isolated from a failed total hip arthroplasty. J Biomed Mater Res B Appl Biomater 2008;86:501–5.
10. Heiner AD, Galvin AL, Fisher J, et al. Scratching vulnerability of conventional vs highly cross-linked polyethylene liners because of large embedded third-body particles. J Arthroplasty 2012;27:742–9.
11. Digas G, Karrholm J, Thanner J, et al. The Otto Aufranc Award. Highly cross-linked polyethylene in total hip arthroplasty: randomized evaluation of penetration rate in cemented and uncemented sockets using radiostereometric analysis. Clin Orthop Relat Res 2004;(429):6–16.
12. Rohrl S, Nivbrant B, Mingguo L, et al. In vivo wear and migration of highly cross-linked polyethylene cups a radiostereometry analysis study. J Arthroplasty 2005;20:409–13.
13. Geller JA, Malchau H, Bragdon C, et al. Large diameter femoral heads on highly cross-linked polyethylene: minimum 3-year results. Clin Orthop Relat Res 2006;447:53–9.
14. Bragdon CR, Greene ME, Freiberg AA, et al. Radiostereometric analysis comparison of wear of highly cross-linked polyethylene against 36- vs 28-mm femoral heads. J Arthroplasty 2007;22:125–9.
15. Ayers DC, Hays PL, Drew JM, et al. Two-year radiostereometric analysis evaluation of femoral head penetration in a challenging population of young total hip arthroplasty patients. J Arthroplasty 2009; 24:9–14.
16. Dorr LD, Wan Z, Shahrdar C, et al. Clinical performance of a Durasul highly cross-linked polyethylene acetabular liner for total hip arthroplasty at five years. J Bone Joint Surg Am 2005;87:1816–21.
17. Engh CA Jr, Stepniewski AS, Ginn SD, et al. A randomized prospective evaluation of outcomes after total hip arthroplasty using cross-linked marathon and non-cross-linked Enduron polyethylene liners. J Arthroplasty 2006;21:17–25.
18. Digas G, Karrholm J, Thanner J, et al. 5-year experience of highly cross-linked polyethylene in cemented and uncemented sockets: two randomized studies using radiostereometric analysis. Acta Orthop 2007;78:746–54.
19. Bragdon CR, Kwon YM, Geller JA, et al. Minimum 6-year followup of highly cross-linked polyethylene in THA. Clin Orthop Relat Res 2007;465:122–7.
20. Kurtz SM, Gawel HA, Patel JD. History and systematic review of wear and osteolysis outcomes for first-generation highly crosslinked polyethylene. Clin Orthop Relat Res 2011;469:2262–77.
21. Mu Z, Tian J, Wu T, et al. A systematic review of radiological outcomes of highly cross-linked polyethylene versus conventional polyethylene in total hip arthroplasty. Int Orthop 2009;33:599–604.
22. Bragdon CR, Doerner M, Martell J, et al. The 2012 John Charnley Award: clinical multicenter studies of the wear performance of highly crosslinked remelted polyethylene in THA. Clin Orthop Relat Res 2013;471:393–402.
23. Dalury DF, Pomeroy DL, Gorab RS, et al. Why are total knee arthroplasties being revised? J Arthroplasty 2013;28:120–1.
24. Lachiewicz PF, Geyer MR. The use of highly cross-linked polyethylene in total knee arthroplasty. J Am Acad Orthop Surg 2011;19:143–51.
25. Jung KA, Lee SC, Hwang SH, et al. Fracture of a second-generation highly cross-linked UHMWPE

tibial post in a posterior-stabilized scorpio knee system. Orthopedics 2008;31:1137.

26. Hermida JC, Fischler A, Colwell CW Jr, et al. The effect of oxidative aging on the wear performance of highly crosslinked polyethylene knee inserts under conditions of severe malalignment. J Orthop Res 2008;26:1585–90.

27. Muratoglu OK, Bragdon CR, Jasty M, et al. Knee-simulator testing of conventional and cross-linked polyethylene tibial inserts. J Arthroplasty 2004;19:887–97.

28. Wang A, Yau SS, Essner A, et al. A highly cross-linked UHMWPE for CR and PS total knee arthroplasties. J Arthroplasty 2008;23:559–66.

29. Utzschneider S, Harrasser N, Schroeder C, et al. Wear of contemporary total knee replacements–a knee simulator study of six current designs. Clin Biomech (Bristol, Avon) 2009;24:583–8.

30. Iwakiri K, Minoda Y, Kobayashi A, et al. In vivo comparison of wear particles between highly crosslinked polyethylene and conventional polyethylene in the same design of total knee arthroplasties. J Biomed Mater Res B Appl Biomater 2009;91:799–804.

31. Hodrick JT, Severson EP, McAlister DS, et al. Highly crosslinked polyethylene is safe for use in total knee arthroplasty. Clin Orthop Relat Res 2008;466:2806–12.

32. Long WJ, Levi GS, Scuderi GR. Highly cross-linked polyethylene in posterior stabilized total knee arthroplasty: early results. Orthop Clin North Am 2012;43:e35–8.

33. Minoda Y, Aihara M, Sakawa A, et al. Comparison between highly cross-linked and conventional polyethylene in total knee arthroplasty. Knee 2009;16:348–51.

34. Wannomae KK, Christensen SD, Micheli BR, et al. Delamination and adhesive wear behavior of alpha-tocopherol-stabilized irradiated ultrahigh-molecular-weight polyethylene. J Arthroplasty 2010;25:635–43.

35. Oral E, Godleski Beckos CA, Lozynsky AJ, et al. Improved resistance to wear and fatigue fracture in high pressure crystallized vitamin E-containing ultrahigh molecular weight polyethylene. Biomaterials 2009;30:1870–80.

36. Haider H, Weisenburger JN, Kurtz SM, et al. Does vitamin E-stabilized ultrahigh-molecular-weight polyethylene address concerns of cross-linked polyethylene in total knee arthroplasty? J Arthroplasty 2012;27:461–9.

Management of Severe Femoral Bone Loss in Revision Total Hip Arthroplasty

Neil P. Sheth, MD[a], Christopher M. Melnic, MD[b],*,
Joshua C. Rozell, MD[b], Wayne G. Paprosky, MD[c]

CrossMark

KEYWORDS

- Revision total hip arthroplasty • Severe femoral bone loss • Preoperative planning • Reconstruction

KEY POINTS

- Femoral bone loss is a complicated problem requiring meticulous preoperative patient evaluation and surgical planning.
- The Paprosky classification system is most commonly used to define femoral bone loss.
- The Paprosky system is based on the location of femoral bone loss, degree of residual proximal femoral bone stock, and the amount of residual isthmus available for diaphyseal fixation.
- More severe bone loss patterns have variable amounts of diaphysis remaining.
- Diaphyseal engaging stems are successful when used with adequate isthmic bone stock. Severe loss of isthmic bone typically requires a cemented option or a megaprosthesis.

BACKGROUND

Total hip arthroplasty (THA) has been shown to be an extremely effective procedure for the treatment of end-stage arthritis of the hip.[1–5] Long-term follow-up continues to demonstrate favorable clinical outcomes[5–9] and as a result, younger, more active patients are being considered candidates for surgery.

Based on the current state of affairs, Kurtz and colleagues[10] have extrapolated the need for THA to increase by more than 170% by 2030. Inherent to this increased utilization of THA is an associated burden of revision surgical procedures. As patient life expectancy continues to increase, THA prostheses are being asked to exhibit improved longevity, which may in turn result in more severe bone loss surrounding the femoral component at the time of revision.

The treatment of femoral bone loss in the setting of revision THA is a challenging problem. This article addresses the etiology of femoral bone loss, associated classification systems, clinical and radiographic patient evaluation, components of effective preoperative planning, and clinical results of various treatment options.

ETIOLOGY OF FEMORAL BONE LOSS

Femoral bone loss may result from osteolysis, stress shielding, periprosthetic infection, periprosthetic fracture, aseptic femoral loosening, iatrogenic bone loss during component removal, and metastatic lesions.[11–13] Regardless of etiology, the pattern of bone loss as well as the degree of residual fixation of the femoral component must be defined preoperatively to determine the appropriate treatment at the time of revision.

The authors have nothing to disclose.
[a] Department of Orthopaedic Surgery, University of Pennsylvania, 800 Spruce Street, 8th Floor Preston Building, Philadelphia, PA 19107, USA; [b] Department of Orthopaedic Surgery, University of Pennsylvania, 3737 Market Street, 6th Floor, Philadelphia, PA 19104, USA; [c] Department of Orthopaedic Surgery, Midwest Orthopaedics, Rush University, 1655 West Harrison Street, Chicago, IL 60612, USA
* Corresponding author.
E-mail address: christopher.melnic@uphs.upenn.edu

Orthop Clin N Am 46 (2015) 329–342
http://dx.doi.org/10.1016/j.ocl.2015.02.002
0030-5898/15/$ – see front matter © 2015 Elsevier Inc. All rights reserved.

FEMORAL BONE LOSS CLASSIFICATIONS

The femoral bone loss classification system proposed by the American Academy of Orthopedic Surgeons is based on the presence of segmental, cavitary, or combined bone defects.[14,15] As has been described previously, the classification system by the American Academy of Orthopedic Surgeons is organized in a simple manner; however, its practical application with regard to the type of treatment that should be used is limited.[15–17]

We advocate the use of the classification system described by Paprosky, which is based on the location of femoral bone loss (metaphyseal or diaphyseal), degree of residual proximal femoral bone stock (ie, amount of cancellous bone loss), and the amount of residual isthmus available for diaphyseal fixation.[15,16] The Paprosky classification system defines 4 different types of femoral bone loss.[18] In type I defects, there is minimal metaphyseal bone loss and the diaphysis is intact. This type of defect is typically not associated with proximal femoral retroversion or varus femoral remodeling (**Fig. 1**). Type II defects, the most commonly encountered pattern, exhibit extensive metaphyseal bone loss with an intact diaphysis. There is a greater degree of proximal femoral remodeling compared with type I femoral defects (**Fig. 2**).

This article focuses on the treatment of more severe bone loss patterns about the femur, specifically types III and IV defects. Type III defects

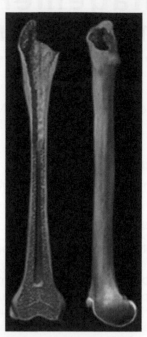

Fig. 2. Type II femoral bone loss. (*Courtesy of* DePuy Synthes, Warsaw, IN.)

exhibit extensive metaphyseal bone loss with some degree of bone loss within the diaphysis. Type III defects are subdivided into types IIIA and IIIB defects. In IIIA defects, there is greater than 4 cm of diaphyseal isthmus remaining, whereas in IIIB defects, there is less than 4 cm of diaphyseal isthmus remaining for femoral component fixation. Theses defects are associated typically with significant proximal femoral remodeling (**Fig. 3**). In type IV defects, there is extensive metadiaphyseal bone loss with complete femoral canal ectasia. The femoral diaphysis is unsupportive and owing to this severe degree of bone loss, there is minimal proximal femoral remodeling (**Fig. 4**).

RADIOGRAPHIC AND CLINICAL PATIENT EVALUATION
Preoperative Planning: Imaging Options

Plain radiographs, including an anteroposterior view of the pelvis and anteroposterior and frog-leg lateral views of the femur (ensuring that the entire length of the existing femoral stem is visible) are usually sufficient to identify the location and severity of femoral bone loss. If there is any concern for femoral deformity (ie, prior ipsilateral total knee arthroplasty, history of infection or congenital deformity, previous femoral fracture) full-length x-rays of the femur can be helpful. Preoperative CT could be obtained to better define the location and severity of femoral bone loss as an adjunct to plain radiographs.[14,19,20]

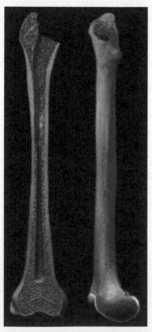

Fig. 1. Type I femoral bone loss. (*Courtesy of* DePuy Synthes, Warsaw, IN.)

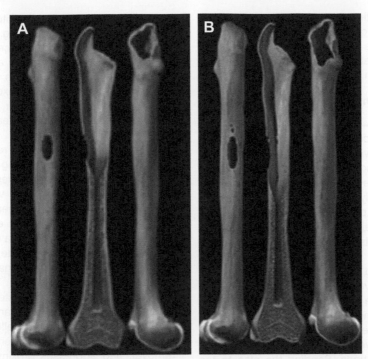

Fig. 3. Type IIIA (*A*) and IIIB (*B*) femoral bone loss. (*Courtesy of* DePuy Synthes, Warsaw, IN.)

Preoperative Planning: Clinical Patient Evaluation

A thorough preoperative patient assessment is critical before femoral component revision. The patient history must document the location, type,

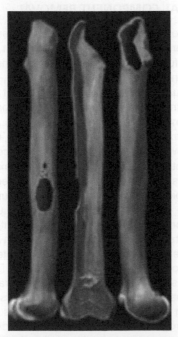

Fig. 4. Type IV femoral bone loss defect. (*Courtesy of* DePuy Synthes, Warsaw, IN.)

character, duration, temporal nature, and exacerbating and remitting factors (ie, activity-related symptoms) of the pain. In addition, a history of all prior procedures and perioperative complications should be recorded.

The lack of a pain-free interval after primary THA prompts questioning of the surgical indication or may indicate low-grade sepsis.[21,22] A diagnosis of deep infection must be ruled out before revision surgery. An erythrocyte sedimentation rate (normal <20 mg/dL) and C-reactive protein (<10 mg/dL) should always be obtained preoperatively and, if elevated, a preoperative hip aspiration should be performed. Synovial fluid obtained from the hip aspiration should routinely be sent for cell count analysis (including differential) and cultures (aerobic and anaerobic). The surgeon must consider the presence of an infection if there are more than 1700 white blood cells in the sample and a differential of greater than 65% segmented neutrophils, if the aspiration is performed outside of the immediate postoperative period.[23,24]

A detailed physical examination includes an assessment of the patient's general health, the lumbosacral spine, contralateral limb, and thorough examination of the affected hip and lower extremity. Assessment of previous incisions about the hip may govern the planned operative approach. A detailed motor, sensory, and vascular examination must also be performed. The patient's gait should be evaluated for the presence of painful ambulation (antalgic gait) and presence of compensatory gait patterns (ie, Trendelenburg gait). Leg lengths should also be evaluated to address appropriately a discrepancy at the time of femoral revision.

Preoperative Planning: Formulating a Detailed Operative Plan

A comprehensive preoperative plan is important for every case; however; it is critical for revision THA where femoral bone loss is present. Several alternate operative plans must be constructed to address adequately unforeseen scenarios encountered during the procedure. Obtaining previous operative reports allows for a better understanding of the components in place and prior operative events.

We recommend the formulation of a detailed, written preoperative plan, which should be distributed to the entire surgical team (**Table 1**). The process of creating this preoperative plan is an extremely effective exercise and allows the surgeon to preemptively prepare for possible intraoperative complications. Sending the plan to the entire surgical team (eg, scrub technician, circulating nurse, anesthesia team, and manufacturing company representatives) minimizes the time spent intraoperatively waiting for instruments and implants (**Box 1**). In addition, identifying items that may be required for addressing potential complications should be set aside preoperatively and made available when needed.

In the academic setting, complex revision cases are often thought of as possessing little educational value, especially for junior residents or residents who do not plan to pursue a fellowship in adult reconstruction. However, detailed preoperative plans present a road map for the case and allow even novice residents to be engaged in the operative procedure (**Box 2**).

SURGICAL APPROACH

The 2 most essential factors when deciding which surgical approach to use for revision femoral surgery are the planned construct for reconstruction and the preference of the attending surgeon. Surgical approach may be influenced by the presence of previous incisions about the hip, although the hip can tolerate multiple incisions without compromising the blood flow to the skin and soft tissues owing to vascular redundancy and robust proximal anastomoses. Selection of the surgical approach is also affected by the location and severity of bone loss (eg, posterior column bone loss prompting the use of a posterior approach), the necessity of an osteotomy, the presence of abnormal anatomy (eg, heterotopic ossification), and unique individual factors (eg, high risk of instability prompting an anterior-based approach). For most complex revisions, we advocate for the posterolateral approach, the most common approach, because it affords excellent acetabular and femoral exposure. However, the surgeon must take into consideration the increased rate of postoperative hip instability.[25–27]

When performing complex revision THA with severe femoral bone loss, having a comprehensive understanding of the osteotomies that can be performed to allow for adequate visualization, safe removal of existing components, and proper reconstruction of the femur is essential. Several osteotomies that should be in a revision THA surgeon's armamentarium include standard single plane, Wagner (anterior), trochanteric slide, and extended trochanteric.[28]

The most commonly used osteotomy in revision THA is the extended trochanteric osteotomy (ETO). This unique osteotomy allows for adequate acetabular exposure, aids in femoral component removal, and addresses proximal femoral varus remodeling by allowing direct access to the remaining diaphysis (**Fig. 5**).[29,30] The use of an ETO in femoral revision THA has demonstrated favorable clinical results. At a mean follow-up of 2.6 years, Paprosky and Sporer reported a 98% union rate of an ETO when used in the setting of revision THA.[29]

FEMORAL COMPONENT REMOVAL

During formulation of a preoperative plan, radiographs and other advanced imaging must be studied carefully to identify key structures that are at risk during implant removal. In addition, the surgeon must have implants available that may be needed in the event that there is a discrepancy between anticipated and actual bone loss encountered intraoperatively. To facilitate stem removal, the following instruments should be accessible: manufacturer-specific explant tools, flexible osteotomes, trephines, high-speed burrs (eg, pencil tip, carbide tip, metal cutting wheel), ultrasonic cement removal instruments, and universal extraction tools that allow attachment to the stem or taper.[31] The surgeon must weigh the risks and benefits of removing a well-fixed acetabular or femoral component.[32]

In the setting of extracting loose femoral stems, it remains important to remove fibrous tissue surrounding the shoulder of the prosthesis to minimize iatrogenic bone loss (**Fig. 6**). Inadvertently trying to remove a stem without clearing the shoulder of the prosthesis may result in additional bone

Table 1
Preoperative patient demographics for the surgical and anesthesia teams

Patient Name: XXXXXX	*Diagnosis: Right Periprosthetic Femoral Fracture*
Age: XXXXXX	*Date of Surgery:* XXXXXX
PMHX: XXXXXX	*Anticoagulation:* ASA 325 mg PO BID × 6 wk
PSHx: R THA	*Post-Pain Mgmt:* Oxycontin 10 mg bid, Celebrex 200 mg PO BID + neurontin 100 mg PO BID
Allergies: XXXXXX	*Implants:* SL revision stem, distal femoral locking plate
Meds: XXXXXX	*Planned Procedure:* Revision right femoral stem/ORIF with prophylactic distal plating/ possible proximal femoral replacement

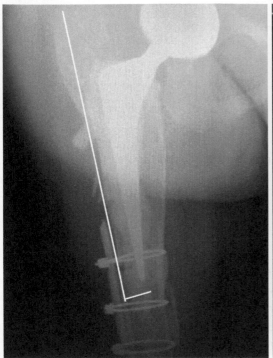 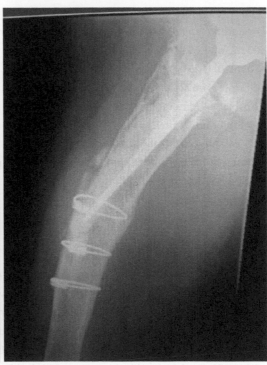

Hbg: x	*K⁺:* x	*BMI:* x	*Cr:* x	*INR:* x	*Albumin:* x

Preop ESR: x	*Pre-op hsCRP:* x

Preop cross-match for 2 units PRBCs

Physical examination:

- Previous posterolateral approach right hip
- Neurovascular intact

Current implants:

Acetabulum: Zimmer continuum 50 cup	*Femur:* Zimmer CPT cemented Stem/32+7

Abbreviations: ASA, aspirin; BID, twice daily; BMI, body mass index; CPT, current procedure terminology; Cr, creatinine; EST, erythrocyte sedimentation rate; Hbg, hemoglobin; hsCRP, highly sensitive C-reactive protein; INR, International Normalized Ratio; Mgmt, management; ORIF, open reduction internal fixation; PO, orally; PRBC, packed red blood cells; PSHx, past surgical history; R, right; THA, total hip arthroplasty.

Box 1
Detailed list of equipment that should be given to operating room staff[a] before the case

Patient position: Lateral decubitus

Table: Radiolucent Jackson table

Positioners: Mizuoki hip positioners

C-arm

Bovie setting: 60/60

Cell saver

Epinephrine soaked sponges

Retractors/special equipment:

- Self-retainer ×2
- Hibbs retractor ×2
- Anaerobic and aerobic culture tissue ×2 specimen cups
- 60 mL of 0.25% Marcaine with epinephrine
- 30 mL of 0.25% Marcaine without epinephrine
- Charnley retractor – *shallow blades*
- 2 proximal femoral elevators (Dark and Stormy)
- #5 Ethibond sutures × 5 + free needles × 2
- #2, #4 and #7 *ZIMMER* acetabular retractors
- Footed impactor, curved curettes, curved osteotomes, bone tamp, and Cobb elevator
- Broad flat osteotome set
- Ball spike pusher
- Anspach - *Pencil tip burr*
- Microsagittal saw
- *DEPUY* Moreland cement removal set
- *BIOMET* Ultradrive for cement removal *(have available but do not open)*
- *BIOMET* Arcos STS stem (190/250 mm length) *(have available but do not open)*
- *ZIMMER* Continuum shell trial liners (50/36) neutral and elevated lip
- *ZIMMER* SL revision femoral stem (length 190 and 265 available)
- *ZIMMER* long-stem CPT (length 240) *(have available but do not open)*
- *SYNTHES* distal femoral locking plate with locking attachment outrigger
- *SYNTHES* cable plate attachments *(have available but do not open)*
- 5 Dall miles cables
- 16 gauge cardiac wire *(have available but do not open)*
- Fibular allograft strut graft *(have available but do not open)*
- Large cement restrictor *(have available but do not open)*

Preoperative Antibiotics: Ancef 2 g IV + Vancomycin 1 g IV.

Abbreviation: IV, intravenous.
  [a] Includes the circulating nurse, scrub technician, and manufacturing representatives.

---

loss or fracture of the greater trochanter. Loose femoral components—most commonly loose cemented stems—also exhibit some degree of proximal remodeling into varus and retroversion (ie, proximal femoral remodeling), which should be recognized preoperatively and the surgical plan should address this deformity.[30]

Recognizing the potential for proximal remodeling preoperatively minimizes the risk of cortical perforation, intraoperative fracture, and

Box 2
A detailed preoperative plan, a roadmap of the planned procedure, for fellows, residents and medical students

Surgical Approach: Extensile posterolateral approach

1. Posterior incision
2. Clearly identify fascia (1 cm in anterior and posterior direction)
3. Fascial incision with curved Mayo scissors
4. Define plane between the underlying g. maximus and deep g. medius
5. Split g. maximus and place Charnley retractor with shallow blades
6. Identify the posterior border of the vastus lateralis → find the g. maximus expansion on the femur
7. Use the bovie to transect the g. max insertion (full thickness)
8. Follow posterior border of the vastus lateralis proximally into a posterior capsular approach
9. Extend the approach proximally over the border of the acetabulum and over the posterior ilium after the posterior border of the gluteus medius
10. Tag the posterior capsule with #5 Ethibond suture on backhand x 3
11. Send *pseudocapsule tissue for final microbiology* × 2 specimen cups
12. Place a Hibbs retractor deep to the g. medius and remove scar tissue anterior to the femoral neck
13. Dislocate the hip once adequate scar tissue has been removed and remove the femoral head

Femoral component removal:

1. Place 2 Dark and Stormy retractors for femoral exposure
2. Clear the shoulder of the prosthesis
3. Release the anterior capsular tether to the proximal femur
4. Remove the cemented CPT stem → should tap out of the cement
5. Extend incision distally to identify the allograft
6. Remove the first 2 cables and the allograft
7. Use the microsaggital saw to perform an ETO of the proximal femoral fracture fragment
8. *Osteotomy length – make osteotomy at level of second wire*
9. Broad osteotomes to open the osteotomy
10. Use the Anspach pencil tip burr to disrupt the cement–prosthesis interface
11. Remove the remainder of the cement within the proximal femur
12. May need *BIOMET* Ultradrive to remove cement under direct visualization
13. Use the 4.5-mm cement drill to penetrate the distal cement plug if needed
14. Use the larger cement drills to drill a larger hole in the cement plug if needed
15. Use back scrapers to try and remove the cement plug and all remaining cement
16. Debride the canal thoroughly

Acetabular component removal:

1. Obtain circumferential exposure of the acetabulum
2. Place #2 and #7 retractors in place for acetabular exposure
3. Remove the liner – size 4.5 mm Synthes screw for liner removal
4. Insert a new a 50/36 trial liner

Femoral reconstruction:

5. Hand ream using the conical *ZIMMER* SL revision tapered reamers → ream under Fluoro
6. Place a trial stem → most likely 265 mm in length → check intra-op fluoro
7. Check hip stability with trial
8. If sizing of the stem is acceptable, then open the real stem and complete reconstruction

9. 3–4 cables for ETO fixation

Distal femoral plating:

1. Make an incision distally for insertion of a distal femoral locking plate
2. Place a K-wire distally
3. Achieve plate balance and place a K-wire proximally distal to the stem
4. Place a screw distally in the metaphysis
5. Place a screw as proximal as possible
6. Place additional screws for fixation
7. Place cables through the proximal incision around the plate and the distal part of the stem
8. Obtain final C-arm images and final flat plate x-rays on the table before complete wound closure

Wound closure:

9. Size 10 flat JP drain × 1 deep to the fascia → (*deep drain distal*)
10. #1 Vicryl × 2 for fascia closure
11. Size 10 flat JP drain × 1 superficial to the fascia → (*superficial drain superior*)
12. #1 Vicryl for deep closure and 2-0 Vicryl for dermal closure
13. 2-0 Nylon suture for the skin – horizontal mattress formation
14. Sterile size 14-inch and 10-inch Aquacel dressings

Postoperative management:

1. TDWB right LE
2. Posterior hip precautions
3. No active abduction × 6 weeks
4. Abduction brace (patient has been called and asked to bring brace from home)
5. ASA 325 mg PO BID × 6 weeks
6. Ancef 1 g q8 hours until intra-op cultures are final
7. Drains to be left in until low output – less than 15 mL/shift

Abbreviations: ASA, aspirin; ETO, extended trochanteric osteotomy; LE, lower extremity; PO, orally; TDWB, touch down weight bearing.

undersizing of the implant. The use of an ETO as an adjunct for exposure can be very useful, particularly in the setting of significant varus remodeling, removal of a well-fixed uncemented implant, or

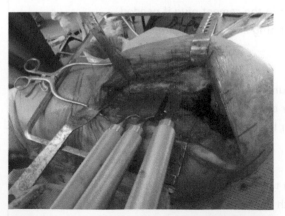

Fig. 5. Intraoperative use of an extended trochanteric osteotomy.

extraction of a long column of cement distal to the stem.[30]

TREATMENT OPTIONS AND CLINICAL OUTCOMES FOR SPECIFIC BONE DEFECTS

The goals of femoral revision are to restore hip biomechanics (ie, restoration of the hip center of rotation, femoral offset, and leg length) and to obtain rotational and axial component stability, while achieving a reconstruction that does not exhibit postoperative instability. In general, biologic fixation of implants is preferred, making cementless devices more commonly used in revision THA surgery. However, there are certain clinical scenarios that require the use of cemented implants.

Type I Defects

The quality and quantity of proximal bone stock, as well as the presence of a loose femoral component

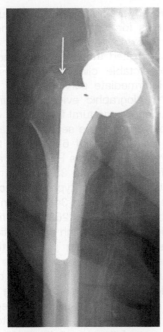

Fig. 6. Anteroposterior hip radiograph with an arrow demonstrating the shoulder of the femoral component with trochanteric overgrowth.

drive the magnitude of proximal femoral remodeling.[30] In type I defects, there is virtually no proximal remodeling and the diaphysis is intact; therefore, a proximally porous coated femoral stem is the reconstruction option of choice. Proximal fitting modular stems (ie, SROM) or extensively porous coated stems may also be used, depending on surgeon preference and the degree of retroversion that is present from proximal femoral remodeling. The design of the SROM allows the metaphysis to be tailored accurately to match the proximal sleeve, and the degree of anteversion can be dialed into the stem independent of the proximal metaphysis. Several studies have demonstrated favorable clinical results with this type of bone loss pattern.[15,16]

Type II Defects

Type II defects are managed typically with 6-inch, extensively porous, coated stems with promising clinical outcomes.[15,16,33] In 1 midterm follow-up study using this type of stem, patients with type II and IIIA defects (133 hips) had only a 5% failure rate.[15] One of the attractions of noncemented femoral stems is the ability to achieve initial diaphyseal fixation. Several types of stems have been used, including fully porous coated stems and dual tapered diaphyseal press fit stems. In a biomechanical study comparing initial fixation of

dual-tapered femoral stems with a rectangular versus a cylindrical cross-section, the rectangular cross-section stems were found to demonstrate superior stability. The cylindrical stems were found to depend on the proximal metaphyseal bone stock whereas the rectangular stems maintained greater stability in the presence of simulated severe proximal bone loss of up to 105 mm.[34]

Type IIIA Defects

Type IIIA defects are defined as having significant proximal remodeling with greater than or equal to 4 cm of isthmus remaining and an absent proximal metaphysis. These defects are typically reconstructed using an extensively porous coated stem or a modular tapered stem. Chung and colleagues[35] performed 96 revisions for 89 type IIIA defects and 7 type IIIB defects. Mean canal diameter was 16.5 mm. At a mean follow-up of 65.7 months, 92 stems achieved bony ingrowth. They concluded that this stem provided good midterm durability.

Sporer and Paprosky[36] evaluated 51 patients with type III or IV defects revised with an extensively porous coated stem for a mean of 4.2 years. A total of 17 patients (33%) were classified as having type IIIA femoral defects. An additional 26 patients (51%) were categorized as having type IIIB defects and 15 (29%) as having a canal diameter of less than 19 mm. There were no failures in the type IIIA defect group and only 1 failure (6.7%) in the type IIIB defect with a canal diameter of less than 19 mm. Patients with type IIIB group and a canal diameter of greater than 19 mm exhibited an 18% failure rate. The authors concluded that extensively porous coated stems should be used for type IIIA defects and for canals less than 19 mm in diameter. Modular tapered stems should be reserved for type IIIB defects and canals with a diameter of greater than 19 mm.

Fluted modular tapered stems have also been evaluated by Park and colleagues[37] At 4.2 years, of the 60% type IIIA and 31% type IIIB defects, none of the patients required additional surgical intervention for mechanical failure at the time of final follow-up.

Type IIIB Defects

Type IIIB defects exhibit extensive metaphyseal bone loss with less than 4 cm of diaphyseal isthmus remaining for femoral fixation. To address this challenging problem, modular tapered, fluted, cementless, distally fixated, porous, titanium stems have gained popularity over the past several years.[38] This stem has become the new "workhorse" for femoral reconstruction. By bypassing the deficient proximal femur and off-loading this unsupported region, forces are transmitted to the diaphysis resulting in eventual biologic fixation.[39]

Modular tapered stems have splines along the length of the disphyseal segment of the prosthesis, which allow for rotational stability (**Fig. 7**). The distal tapered geometry is able to engage a short isthmic segment more effectively than a stem with cylindrical distal geometry and can satisfy the 2 to 3 cm of diaphyseal contact required for stability.[40] Additionally, the modulus of elasticity of titanium is similar to that of bone, which may minimize modulus mismatch and thus decrease thigh pain and stress shielding.

When the anatomy of the lesser trochanter is altered through femoral remodeling or there is severe proximal bone loss that includes the lesser trochanter, judging the appropriate version of the stem can be challenging. Modular tapered stems provide the flexibility to adjust femoral version independent of the diaphyseal segment of the component, allowing for optimal THA stability.[40] The proximal body facilitates control of anteversion, offset, and leg length, thus restoring native hip biomechanics. Allowing the proximal body trial to rotate on a well-fixed distal segment during trial reduction facilitates appropriate anteversion, which in turn decreases the risk of postoperative dislocation.[41,42] The surgeon also has the ability to correct leg length discrepancies by intraoperatively fine tuning the length of the proximal body. In addition, the proximal body of a modular tapered stem may exhibit host bone contact with the remaining metaphysis and result in supplemental implant to bone healing or biologic fixation.

In a study by Palumbo and colleagues,[41] 211 revision THAs for type III and IV femoral bone loss were followed over an average of 4.5 years. They demonstrated that modular tapered stems provide predictable clinical outcomes and an excellent intermediate survivorship of 94%. No clinical or radiographic evidence of implant or modular junction structural failure was observed. Comparable results were seen in 58 patients followed for an average of 67 months to assess osseous integration, Harris Hip Score, and survivorship of the implant. In 33 patients with type IIIB defects and 25 with type IV defects, Harris Hip Score improved from 34 to 74 on average, with 15 of 58 patients (26%) experiencing a complication. Despite a high complication rate in this subset of challenging patients, there was 98% implant survivorship overall.[38]

Early studies focused their evaluation on the use of a single nonmodular stem. Grünig and colleagues[43] evaluated 38 revisions and reported an 8% (3/38) rate of re-revision owing to stem subsidence by mean follow-up of 47 months. Isacson and colleagues[44] evaluated 43 hips treated with a single nonmodular stem at a mean follow-up of 25 months. Although almost all patients demonstrated abundant new bone formation, 5 of 42 patients (12%) had subsidence of greater than 20 mm and 22 (52%) had subsidence of less than 5 mm.

Several studies have evaluated clinical outcome scores in patients treated with modular versus nonmodular stems. Richards and colleagues and Garbuz and colleagues reported superior results with modular tapered femoral components. Despite modular stems being used in cases with more severe bone loss (65% Paprosky types IIIB and IV femurs vs 35% in the nonmodular group), quality of life scores were higher, there were fewer intraoperative fractures, and there was increased reestablishment of host bone compared with nonmodular stems.[31,45,46] Owing to the subpar results demonstrated with the use of a nonmodular stem in comparison with the results seen with a modular stem, we support the use of modular stems when addressing severe femoral bone loss defects.

Type IV Defects

Managing type IV femoral bone loss is a major challenge for the revision hip arthroplasty surgeon. Treatment for type IV defects usually involves the use of a cemented stem with or without impaction bone grafting, allograft prosthesis composite (APC) reconstruction, or the use of a proximal femoral replacement megaprosthesis. In this setting, extensively porous coated or modular tapered stems are

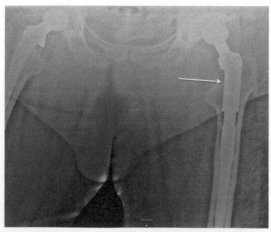

Fig. 7. Anteroposterior hip radiograph with an arrow demonstrating the proximal body of a modular tapered stem.

ineffective typically owing to the lack of femoral isthmus remaining for diaphyseal fixation.

Indications for impaction grafting include significant osteolysis or stress shielding where the femoral canal is enlarged with a so-called stove pipe appearance (>18 mm in diameter) and the length of the intact diaphysis is inadequate to achieve an interference fit for a cementless implant.[47] To impact the bone chips, a trial prosthesis mimicking the dimensions of the cemented standard stem is driven into the proximal femur over a central wire. Deficiencies of the femoral cortex should be reinforced with segments of wire mesh. Bone chips no larger than 1 to 2 mm should be added to prevent fractures. Once the canal is filled completely, the real femoral stem is cemented into the neomedullary canal. Of note, it is important to ensure that the cement mantle is at least 2 mm.[48]

High complication rates were encountered in several of the initial studies evaluating impaction grafting. Of their 34 complications in type III and IV defects, Pekkarinen and colleagues[49] described 17 intraoperative fractures of the femoral diaphysis or greater trochanter and 3 cases of subsidence greater than 10 mm. With average follow-up of 30 months in their series of 34 patients, Meding and colleagues[50] reported an intraoperative fracture rate of 12% and a 38% rate of stem subsidence. Given these results, Meding and associates advised that impaction bone grafting only be used if the proximal femoral bone loss was so severe that stability could not be obtained using a long uncemented femoral stem.

The addition of allograft struts in impaction grafting has produced more promising results over recent years. Strut grafts are individually sized beams of nonvital bone attached to the deficient femur via tension bands or cable wires. Incorporation and remodeling of these allografts to the host bone has been shown to be successful in 80% to 100 % of cases.[51] Buttaro and colleagues,[52] in their cohort of 25 hips (14 with type IV and 11 with type IIIB defects), showed that mean femoral width was increased by 41% and overall survivorship was 95% at a mean of 54.5 months. There was no evidence of osteolysis, resorption, or radiolucencies during follow-up in any hip. There were also no infections or dislocations. Here, the combination of intramedullary and extramedullary biological reconstruction with bone allografts and cemented polished tapered stems was associated with favorable survivorship and mechanical stability in patients with severe femoral bone loss.

In one of the largest prospective studies of impaction grafting used to restore bone loss, Gie and colleagues evaluated 540 cases over an average of 6.7 years (range, 2–15). The majority of the 487 patients included in this study underwent revision hip arthroplasty for aseptic loosening (81% of cases). In all but 1 case, the group used a cemented femoral component with morselized cancellous bone graft. There was a 15% complication rate including 29 periprosthetic fractures (5.4%). A total of 494 hips remained successfully in situ at latest follow-up. The 10-year survival rate was 98.0% (95% CI, 96.2–99.8) with aseptic loosening as the endpoint and 84.2% (95% CI, 78.5–89.9) for reoperation for any reason. The authors attributed the complication rate primarily to the difficult and complex nature of the revision surgery rather than the impaction grafting technique.[53]

An additional option is APC reconstruction, an attractive option because of its ability to reattach soft tissues and improve bone stock to facilitate future reconstruction. The current role of an APC is for the treatment of severe proximal metaphyseal bone loss with associated diaphyseal defects that involve bone distal to the isthmus. In this scenario, there is insufficient bone stock to use a distal fixation prosthesis.[54] The APC uses a long stem prosthesis that spans the host–allograft bone junction. When possible, the prosthesis is cemented into the allograft and "press-fit" into the residual host femoral diaphysis.

Blackley and colleagues[55] evaluated 63 APC constructs at a mean follow-up of 11 years. They identified a success rate of 77% for the 45 patients who survived to the latest follow-up. The nonunion rate at the host–graft junction was 6% and other complications included hip instability, deep infection, and aseptic loosening. Nearly 27% of the grafts demonstrated some degree of resorption on x-ray. Loosening of the APC may occur between the cement–implant or cement–allograft interface. Any failure causes shortening of the limb and should be treated with revision. The increased rate of complication here may be owing to the greater technical demands imposed by the surgery itself or patient disease. A metaanalysis evaluating revisions for failed APC reconstructions described 21 patients with a mean follow-up of 170 months. The use of long smooth stems, neither press-fit nor cemented to minimize distal bone damage, demonstrated a 5- and 10-year survival rate of 83.5%. Therefore, an APC reconstruction seems to be a promising option for severe proximal bone loss.[56]

The megaprosthesis or proximal femoral replacement has been used traditionally for limb salvage in the elderly, low-demand patient in whom resection arthroplasty is the only reasonable alternative. Although this construct allows early weight bearing with shorter operative times and does not pose a risk of disease transmission like the APC, there are also several disadvantages. The most commonly reported complication is dislocation, ranging from 8% to 22%.[57–60] Additional complications include early loosening, instability, stress shielding, limb-length discrepancy, and cost.[31]

Haentjens and colleagues[61] evaluated 16 patients, at a mean follow-up of 5 years, treated with the megaprosthesis for failed THA. All patients still required assistive devices for ambulation despite a reduction in pain, and 7 patients suffered a dislocation. More recently, a retrospective review of 15 patients with mean follow-up of 64 months exhibited improvement in Harris Hip Scores from 28 to 69 with 2 dislocations and a mean survivorship of 87% at 5 years.[62] Overall, the use of the megaprosthesis poses several complex and long-term problems and should only be used as a salvage procedure in low-demand patients.

SUMMARY

The treatment of femoral bone loss continues to be a very difficult problem in revision THA. Accurate preoperative bone loss pattern assessment along with formation of a detailed preoperative plan is essential for achieving clinical success. This plan is imperative to understanding the different available treatment options and the clinical scenarios for which each treatment is appropriate. Thorough preoperative planning for a challenging femoral revision case, with all appropriate surgical/technical equipment made available, allows one to avoid excessive thinking in the operating room and for execution of a premeditated plan.

REFERENCES

1. Laupacis A, Bourne R, Rorabeck C, et al. The effect of elective total hip replacement on health-related quality of life. J Bone Joint Surg Am 1993;75: 1619–26.
2. Learmonth I, Young C, Rorabeck C. The operation of the century: total hip replacement. Lancet 2007;370: 1508–19.
3. Charnley J. The long-term results of low-friction arthroplasty of the hip performed as a primary intervention. 1972. Clin Orthop Relat Res 1995;(319):4–15.
4. Khanuja H, Vakil J, Goddard M, et al. Cementless femoral fixation in total hip arthroplasty. J Bone Joint Surg Am 2011;93:500–9.
5. Pivec R, Johnson A, Mears S, et al. Hip arthroplasty. Lancet 2012;380:1768–77.
6. Caton J, Prudhon J. Over 25 years survival after Charnley's total hip arthroplasty. Int Orthop 2011; 35:185–8.
7. Callaghan J, Bracha P, Liu S, et al. Survivorship of a Charley total hip arthroplasty. A concise follow-up, at a minimum of 35 years, of previous reports. J Bone Joint Surg Am 2009;91:2617–21.
8. Hailer N, Garellick G, Karrholm J. Uncemented and cemented primary total hip arthroplasty in the Swedish hip arthroplasty register. Acta Orthop 2010;81:33–41.
9. Rasquinha V, Dua V, Rodriguez J, et al. Fifteen-year survivorship of a collarless, cemented, normalized femoral stem in primary hybrid total hip arthroplasty with a modified third-generation cement technique. J Arthroplasty 2003;18(Suppl 1):86–94.
10. Kurtz S, Ong K, Lau E, et al. Projections of primary and revision hip and knee arthroplasty in the United States from 2005 to 2030. J Bone Joint Surg Am 2007;90:780–5.
11. Clohisy J, Calvert G, Tull F, et al. Reasons for revision hip surgery: a retrospective review. Clin Orthop Relat Res 2004;429:188–92.
12. Dobzyniak M, Fehring T, Odum S. Early failure in total hip arthroplasty. Clin Orthop Relat Res 2006; 447:76–8.
13. Paprosky W, Greidanus N, Antoniou J. Minimum 10-year results of extensively porous-coated stems in revision hip arthroplasty. Clin Orthop Relat Res 1999;(369):230–42.
14. D'Antonio J, McCarthy J, Bargar W, et al. Classification of femoral abnormalities in total hip arthroplasty. Clin Orthop Relat Res 1993;(296):133–9.
15. Paprosky W, Aribindi R. Hip replacement: treatment of femoral bone loss using distal bypass fixation. Instr Course Lect 2000;49:119–30.
16. Pak J, Paprosky W, Jablonsky W, et al. Femoral strut allografts in cementless revision total hip arthroplasty. Clin Orthop Relat Res 1993;(295):172–8.
17. Aribindi R, Barba M, Solomon M, et al. Bypass fixation. Orthop Clin North Am 1998;29:319–29.
18. Paprosky W, Burnett R. Assessment and classification of bone stock deficiency in revision total hip arthroplasty. Am J Orthop 2002;31:459–64.
19. Park J, Ryu K, Hong H, et al. Focal osteolysis in total hip replacement: CT findings. Skeletal Radiol 2004; 33:632–40.
20. Kaltsas D. Infection after total hip arthroplasty. Ann R Coll Surg Engl 2004;86:267–71.
21. Fitzgerald R. Infected total hip arthroplasty: diagnosis and treatment. J Am Acad Orthop Surg 1995;3:249–62.
22. Sakellariou V, Babis G. Management bone loss of the proximal femur in revision hip arthroplasty: update on reconstructive options. World J Orthop 2014;18:614–22.

23. Weeden S, Paprosky W, Bowling J. The early dislocation rate in primary total hip arthroplasty following the posterior approach with posterior soft-tissue repair. J Arthroplasty 2003;18:709–13.

24. Roberts J, Fu F, McClain E, et al. A comparison of the posterolateral and anterolateral approaches to total hip arthroplasty. Clin Orthop Relat Res 1984;(187):205–10.

25. Morrey B. Instability after total hip arthroplasty. Orthop Clin North Am 1992;23:237–48.

26. Ghanem E, Parvizi J, Burnett R, et al. Cell count and differential of aspirated fluid in the diagnosis of infection at the site of total knee arthroplasty. J Bone Joint Surg Am 2008;90:1637–43.

27. Della Valle C, Sporer S, Jacobs J, et al. Preoperative testing for sepsis before revision total knee arthroplasty. J Arthroplasty 2007;22:90–3.

28. Archibeck M, Rosenberg A, Berger R, et al. Trochanteric osteotomy and fixation during total hip arthroplasty. J Am Acad Orthop Surg 2003;11:163–73.

29. Paprosky W, Sporer S. Controlled femoral fracture: easy in. J Arthroplasty 2003;18:91–3.

30. Foran J, Brown N, Della Valle C, et al. Prevalence, risk factors, and management of proximal femoral remodeling in revision hip arthroplasty. J Arthroplasty 2013;28:877–81.

31. Sheth N, Nelson C, Paprosky W. Femoral bone loss in revision total hip arthroplasty: evaluation and management. J Am Acad Orthop Surg 2013;21:601–12.

32. Maloney W, Herzwurm P, Paprosky W, et al. Treatment of pelvic osteolysis associated with a stable acetabular component inserted without cement as part of a total hip replacement. J Bone Joint Surg Am 1997;79:1628–34.

33. Weeden S, Paprosky W. Minimal 11-year follow up of extensively porous-coated stems in femoral revision total hip arthroplasty. J Arthroplasty 2002;17:134–7.

34. Sangorgio S, Ebramzadeh E, Knutsen A, et al. Fixation of non-cemented total hip arthroplasty femoral components in a simulated proximal bone defect model. J Arthroplasty 2013;28:1618–24.

35. Chung L, Wu P, Chen C, et al. Extensively porous-coated stems for femoral revision: reliable choice for stem revision in Paprosky femoral type III defects. Orthopedics 2012;35:1017–21.

36. Sporer S, Paprosky W. Revision total hip arthroplasty: the limitations of fully coated stems. Clin Orthop Relat Res 2003;(417):203–9.

37. Park Y, Moon Y, Lim S. Revision total hip arthroplasty using a fluted and tapered modular distal fixation stem with and without extended trochanteric osteotomy. J Arthroplasty 2007;22:993–9.

38. Brown N, Tetreault M, Cipriano C, et al. Modular tapered implants for severe femoral bone loss in THA: reliable osseointegration but frequent complications. Clin Orthop Relat Res 2015;473:555–60.

39. Rodriguez J, Deshmukh A, Klauser W, et al. Patterns of osseointegration and remodeling in femoral revision with bone loss using modular, tapered, fluted, titanium stems. J Arthroplasty 2011;26:1409–17.

40. Cross M, Paprosky W. Managing femoral bone loss in revision total hip replacement: fluted tapered modular stems. Bone Joint J 2013;95B:95–7.

41. Palumbo B, Morrison K, Baumgarten A, et al. Results of revision total hip arthroplasty with modular, titanium-tapered femoral stems in severe proximal metaphyseal and diaphyseal bone loss. J Arthroplasty 2013;28:690–4.

42. Stimac J, Boles J, Parkes N, et al. Revision total hip arthroplasty with modular femoral stems. J Arthroplasty 2014;29:2167–70.

43. Grünig R, Morscher E, Oschsner P. Three-to 7-year results with the uncemented SL femoral revision prosthesis. Arch Orthop Trauma Surg 1997;116:187–97.

44. Isacson J, Stark A, Wallensten R. The Wagner revision prosthesis consistently restores femoral bone structure. Int Orthop 2000;24:139–42.

45. Garbuz D, Toms A, Masri B, et al. Improved outcome in femoral revision arthroplasty with tapered fluted modular titanium stems. Clin Orthop Relat Res 2006;453:199–202.

46. Richards C, Duncan C, Masri B, et al. Femoral revision hip arthroplasty: a comparison of two stem designs. Clin Orthop Relat Res 2010;468:491–6.

47. Mayle R, Paprosky WG. Massive bone loss: allograft-prosthetic composites and beyond. Bone Joint J 2012;94:61–4.

48. Gehrke T, Gebauer M, Kendoff D. Femoral stem impaction grafting: extending the role of cement. Bone Joint J 2013;95B:92–4.

49. Pekkarinen J, Alho A, Lepistö J, et al. Impaction bone grafting in revision hip surgery: a high incidence of complications. Bone Joint J 2000;82B:103–7.

50. Meding JB, Ritter MA, Keating EM, et al. Impaction bone-grafting before insertion of a femoral stem with cement in revision total hip arthroplasty: a minimum two-year follow-up study. J Bone Joint Surg Am 1997;79A:1834–41.

51. Kinkel S, Thomsen MN, Nadorf J, et al. Strut grafts in revision hip arthroplasty faced with femoral bone defects: an experimental analysis. Int Orthop 2014;38:1147–53.

52. Buttaro MA, Costantini J, Comba F, et al. The use of femoral struts and impacted cancellous bone allograft in patients with severe femoral bone loss who undergo revision total hip replacement: a three- to nine-year follow-up. Bone Joint J 2012;94:167–72.

53. Lamberton T, Kenny P, Whitehouse S, et al. Femoral impaction grafting in revision total hip arthroplasty: a follow-up of 540 hips. J Arthroplasty 2011;26:1154–60.

54. Sternheim A, Rogers BA, Kuzyk PR, et al. Segmental proximal femoral bone loss and revision total hip replacement in patients with developmental dysplasia of the hip: the role of allograft prosthesis composite. Bone Joint J 2012;94:762–7.

55. Blackley HR, Davis AM, Hutchinson CR, et al. Proximal femoral allografts for reconstruction of bone stock in revision arthroplasty of the hip. J Bone Joint Surg Am 2001;83A:346–54.

56. Sternheim A, Drexler M, Kuzyk PR, et al. Treatment of failed allograft prosthesis composites used for hip arthroplasty in the setting of severe proximal femoral bone defects. J Arthroplasty 2014;29: 1058–62.

57. Al-Taki M, Masri B, Duncan CP, et al. Quality of life following proximal femoral replacement using a modular system in revision THA. Clin Orthop Relat Res 2011;469:470–5.

58. Parvizi J, Tarity TD, Slenker N, et al. Proximal femoral replacement in patients with non-neoplastic conditions. J Bone Joint Surg Am 2007;89:1036–43.

59. Zehr R, Enneking W, Scarborough M. Allograft-prosthesis composite versus megaprosthesis in proximal femoral reconstruction. Clin Orthop Relat Res 1996;(322):207–23.

60. Malkani A, Lewallen D, Cabanela M, et al. Femoral component revision using an uncemented, proximally coated, long-stem prosthesis. J Arthroplasty 1996;11: 411–8.

61. Haentjens P, Boeck H, Opdecam P. Proximal femoral replacement prosthesis for salvage of failed hip arthroplasty: complications in a 2–11 year follow-up study in 19 elderly patients. Acta Orthop Scand 1996;67:37–42.

62. Sewell M, Hanna S, Carrington R, et al. Modular proximal femoral replacement in salvage hip surgery for non-neoplastic conditions. Acta Orthop Belg 2010;76:493–502.

Reducing Blood Loss in Bilateral Total Knee Arthroplasty with Patient-Specific Instrumentation

Parthiv A. Rathod, MD[a],*, Ajit J. Deshmukh, MD[b],
Fred D. Cushner, MD[c]

KEYWORDS

- Blood loss • Bilateral knee arthroplasty • Patient-specific instrumentation

KEY POINTS

- The authors found a reduction in combined tourniquet time with the use of patient-specific instrumentation (PSI) in simultaneous bilateral total knee arthroplasty (TKA). Thus, PSI has the potential for better cost efficiency resulting from the reduction in surgical time in addition to the need for fewer numbers of surgical trays.
- Avoidance of instrumentation of the intramedullary canal of the femur can theoretically decrease the blood loss during surgery. The authors found a trend to reduced total blood loss as measured by drop in hemoglobin (Hgb) values after surgery and a trend to lower transfusion rate after surgery.
- The authors did not find any differences in the rate of thromboembolism or early complications with or without the use of PSI.
- Length of stay was lower with the use of PSI in bilateral TKA compared with not using PSI, but it was not statistically significant.
- Further research in the forms of high-quality randomized trials and cost-benefit analyses may help in further consolidation of these findings.

INTRODUCTION
Patient-Specific Instrumentation

The demand for primary TKA has escalated in recent times and is expected to double by 2016.[1] Recent technological advances have, therefore, aimed at improving surgical reproducibility, efficiency, and patient outcomes. One such advancement is the development of PSI. PSI in TKA has been introduced to obtain consistent alignment, prevent instrumentation of the medullary canal, and improve operating room efficiency.[2–4] A preoperative MRI or CT scan of the lower extremity is obtained, which is used by an implant manufacturer to generate a simulated version of a patient's knee anatomy. With the help of specialized software, bony resections and component sizes are planned based on surgeon preferences and patient factors. Custom cutting guides are then fabricated, sterilized, and supplied to the surgeon's hospital, ready for the operating room. Proposed advantages of PSI include consistency of component and limb

Conflict of Interest Statement: The senior author (F.D. Cushner) is a paid consultant and receives royalties from Smith & Nephew. Other authors—no conflicts reported. There was no external funding source for this study.
[a] NYU Hospital for Joint Diseases, Woodhull Hospital, NYU Langone Medical Center, New York, NY, USA; [b] VA New York Harbor Healthcare System, NYU Hospital for Joint Diseases, NYU Langone Medical Center, New York, NY, USA; [c] Southside Hospital, North Shore LIJ Health System, New York, NY, USA
* Corresponding author. Department of Surgery Administration, 760 Broadway, Brooklyn, NY 11206.
E-mail address: drparthivrathod@gmail.com

alignment, avoidance of intramedullary instrumentation, potential for improved patient outcomes, and better cost efficiency resulting from a decrease in the number of surgical trays and reduced surgical time and operating room turnover time. Theoretically, avoidance of intramedullary instrumentation may result in reduced blood loss (and therefore transfusion requirement) as well as decreased risk of systemic embolization, which ultimately has the potential to reduce inpatient length of stay (LOS), another potential cost savings for the hospital. The added cost of imaging and fabrication of patient-specific guides is, however, a concern.

Many previous studies have compared alignment obtained with PSI and standard instrumentation, with mixed results.[4–16] Fewer investigators have studied the influence of PSI on surgical time, blood loss, and LOS.[6–9,13,16–20] Some studies have demonstrated a small but significant reduction in surgical time,[7,8,13] whereas some studies did not.[6,9,17] Similarly, there seems to be no consensus on whether there is truly an advantage of reduced blood loss, transfusion requirements, and LOS.[7,8,13,16] No study has specifically compared surgical time, blood loss, transfusion requirements, and LOS associated with PSI in simultaneous bilateral TKA with a control group of non-PSI bilateral TKA.

Study Aims

A retrospective comparative study was performed to assess surgical time and compare early results after simultaneous bilateral TKA with and without the use of PSI, by the same surgeon and using the same implant system. The authors specifically compared 2 groups of patients evaluating (1) surgical time, (2) blood loss and transfusion requirements, (3) inpatient LOS and, lastly, (4) early thromboembolic events and complication rate.

METHODS

Institutional board approval was obtained for this study. The authors retrospectively reviewed the office charts, operating room notes, and medical records of all patients undergoing simultaneous bilateral TKAs by a single surgeon at 2 institutions from April 2011 through February 2012. Twenty-nine patients (58 TKAs) formed the study cohort. The authors included all patients undergoing simultaneous bilateral TKA during this time frame and no patients were excluded.

The senior surgeon, Dr. Cushner started using PSI for TKA in April 2011. The decision to offer PSI versus conventional instrumentation was based entirely on the surgeon's discretion. Based on whether PSI had been used or not, 2 patient groups were formed (**Table 1**). The non-PSI group

Table 1
Patient groups

PSI	Non-PSI
15 Patients/30 knees	14 Patients/28 knees
6 Men/9 women, mean age 57 y (Mean [SD] 4.5)	6 Men/8 women, mean age 59 y (Mean [SD] 6.5)
Legion (Smith & Nephew) TKA with Visionaire	Legion (Smith & Nephew) TKA with standard instrumentation and OrthAlign for tibial cut

included 14 patients (28 knees). This group comprised 8 women and 6 men, with a mean age of 59 years (Mean [SD] 6.5) and mean body mass index (BMI) of 29 (Mean [SD] 4.5). The PSI group consisted of 15 patients (30 knees) with 9 women and 6 men, having a mean age of 57 years (Mean [SD] 6.6) and mean BMI of 30 (Mean [SD] 5.1). Preoperative diagnosis was osteoarthritis in all knees.

All patients received a similar design of posterior-stabilized cemented TKA by the same manufacturer. All surgeries were performed using either the Legion or Journey II posterior-stabilized TKA standard instrumentation with OrthAlign for tibial cut in non-PSI group system (Smith & Nephew, Memphis, Tennessee) and the Visionaire (Smith & Nephew) PSI was used in PSI group. The latter is an MRI-based PSI system, which, in addition to the MRI, uses long-leg radiographs for preoperative planning.

Patients donated 2 units of autologous blood and were given 3 erythropoetin injections (40,000 IU each) (Procrit, Centocor Ortho Biotech, Horsham, Pennsylvania), 3 weeks, 2 weeks, and 1 week prior to surgery. All patients received oral sustained-release oxycodone (20 mg) (OxyContin, Purdue Pharma, Stamford, Connecticut) and celecoxib (200 mg) (Celebrex, Pfizer, New York, New York) preemptively.

Spinal anesthesia was given to all patients followed by bilateral femoral nerve blocks. A pneumatic tourniquet set to 300 mm Hg to 350 mm Hg (based on body habitus) was used in all cases and was inflated prior to skin incision and deflated after skin closure and application of compression dressing.

A medial parapatellar arthrotomy was used for exposure. In the non-PSI group, a handheld accelerometer-based surgical navigation system (KneeAlign, OrthAlign, Aliso Viejo, California) was used to make the tibial resection first, followed by distal femoral resection using a conventional intramedullary alignment rod. The handheld navigation was not used for femoral resection. The remaining femoral cuts were performed after setting the femoral rotation based on the transepicondylar axis and Whiteside line. The femoral canal was capped in all non-PSI cases with a bone plug made from resected bone. In the PSI group, all femoral cuts were performed first as recommended by the manufacturer and tibial resection was performed last using the fabricated guides. Osteophyte removal and soft tissue releases were performed to balance flexion-extension gaps. Patella resurfacing was performed in all knees. Closure was performed over a deep reinfusion drain, which was clamped for the first 4 hours and removed on postoperative day (POD) 1. Blood was reinfused if the output was more than 100 mL in the first 6 hours after unclamping of drains. Closure was performed using knotless barbed sutures (Quill Self-Retaining System, Angiotech Pharmaceuticals, Vancouver, British Columbia, Canada), using #2 for closure of the arthrotomy, #0 for the subcutaneous layer, and #2-0 for subcuticular closure.

A sterile compression dressing was then applied and compression maintained for 24 hours. Cryotherapy was initiated. Postoperatively, patients received short- and long-acting oral oxycodone, acetaminophen, and celecoxib, with intravenous morphine as needed. Patients were encouraged to get out of bed on POD1 and active and passive knee range-of-motion exercises were initiated. Subcutaneous enoxaparin injections were used for thromboembolism prophylaxis starting 18 to 24 hours after surgery and continued for 2 weeks postoperatively. The criteria for blood transfusion were standardized and included either presence of signs or symptoms of anemia or hypovolemia unresponsive to fluid resuscitation or Hgb concentration less than 7.5 g/dL. Complete blood cell count was performed daily for the first 3 days of inpatient stay and then as needed. Physical therapy was provided daily, starting POD1. Patients were allowed full weight bearing with a walker frame. According to the prespecified home discharge criteria set forth by the 2 hospitals, patients were allowed to go home if they were able to walk 150 feet (46 m), independently transfer from a bed and chair, and go up and down a flight of stairs. Patients were discharged to a skilled nursing facility if they failed to meet the discharge to home criteria. Social work was consulted on POD1 to facilitate eventual discharge.

Tourniquet time was evaluated as a measure of the length of the surgical procedure. Tourniquet time was added for the 2 sides to generate the total tourniquet time. The reduction in Hgb concentration was used as a measure of blood loss and was calculated based on serial postoperative Hgb levels using preoperative Hgb (obtained just prior to surgery) as baseline. Blood transfusion rates were analyzed and compared between groups. Inpatient LOS was assessed in days with the day after surgery counted as the first day and the day of discharge counted as the last day. All thromboembolic episodes were noted up to 3 months postoperatively. Similarly, all early reoperations and complications were noted.

Data were analyzed to determine if there was a significant difference between the 2 groups in demographics, preoperative and postoperative Hgb values, maximum Hgb reduction, average number of allogeneic units transfused in the 2 groups, tourniquet time, LOS, and disposition. Independent t tests were used for comparing continuous data and chi-square test (with Fisher exact test) for comparing categorical data. The level of statistical significance was set at $P = .05$. Statistical analyses were performed using SPSS, Version 16, software (Chicago, Illinois).

OUTCOMES

Both groups were comparable in terms of patient demographics, such as age ($P = .7$), gender ($P = .53$), and BMI ($P = .5$) (**Table 2**). Although the PSI group started off with a lower preoperative Hgb concentration, this was statistically comparable ($P = .5$) between groups. Intraoperatively, all custom blocks were found to have acceptable fit and accuracy, and no PSI procedures had to be abandoned or modified. Surgical time, as indicated by total tourniquet time, for bilateral TKAs combined was 18 minutes lower in PSI group (mean 123.6 minutes 13.4 [SD]) compared with the non-PSI group (mean 141.1 minutes 13.9 [SD]) ($P = .001$). There was a trend for lower Hgb drop in the PSI group (mean [SD] = 2.87 [1.5]) compared with the non-PSI group (mean [SD] = 4.03 [2]; $P = .07$). The average units of allogeneic blood transfused were lower in the PSI group (trend, $P = .1$). LOS was lower in the PSI group but not statistically significant ($P = .16$). All patients in this study were discharged to a skilled nursing facility.

COMPLICATIONS

There were no cases of pulmonary embolism (PE) in the study cohort. One patient in PSI group, however, underwent PE screening, which included chest radiograph, electrocardiogram, bilateral lower extremity Doppler, and CT angiography for clinical suspicion of PE. In each group, 1 patient developed unilateral deep venous thrombosis (DVT). One knee in PSI group underwent

Table 2
Outcome parameters in study groups, mean (SD)

Group	Preoperative Hemoglobin	Postoperative Day 1 Hemoglobin	Postoperative Day 2 Hemoglobin	Postoperative Day 3 Hemoglobin	Minimum Hemoglobin	Maximum Hemoglobin Difference	Allogeneic Transfusion (Units)	Tourniquet Time	Length of Stay
PSI group	12.1 (1.6)	10.2 (1.0)	9.8 (1.2)	9.7 (0.7)	9.2 (1.0)	2.87 (1.5)	0.5 (0.7)	123.6 (13.4)	3.9 (1.4)
Non-PSI group	12.8 (1.6)	10.7 (1.0)	9.6 (1.0)	9.2 (1.1)	8.8 (0.9)	4.03 (2)	1.2 (1.8)	141.9 (13.9)	5 (2.0)
P value	.5	.5	.2	.1	.2	.07[a]	.1[a]	.001[b]	.16

[a] Trend.
[b] Significant value.

reoperation for a deep hematoma, with irrigation, débridement, and reclosure of the incision. The prevalence of postoperative stiffness necessitating manipulation under anesthesia (MUA) was 2 patients in PSI group compared with 2 patients in the non-PSI group and hence was similar between groups (**Table 3**).

DISCUSSION
Surgical Time

The use of PSI in simultaneous bilateral TKA in the authors' study resulted in reduced total tourniquet time (**Table 4**). This reduction in tourniquet time seems consistent with some previous reports.[5–8,13,21] As suggested by some investigators, this finding may be a result of reduced number of surgical steps with the PSI system. Some other studies, however, were unable to demonstrate an advantage in surgical times with the PSI system.[9,17] This may be due to a difference in surgical techniques, surgeon volume, experience with custom blocks, and inherent differences in PSI of different manufacturers. Previous studies have indicated that the cost benefits of faster surgical time may not be significant to outweigh the increased cost of additional preoperative imaging and custom blocks.[5] Duffy suggested that this reduction in operating room time may cumulatively help surgeons perform increased number of surgical procedures.[2]

Blood Loss and Length of Stay

Decreased blood loss is another factor that can improve outcomes and cost effectiveness after TKA. In this study, the authors found a trend to lower blood loss in the PSI group compared with the non-PSI group. Number of units transfused again were lower with PSI but did not reach statistical significance. Some studies investigating the use of PSI in unilateral TKA have found small (100 mL) but significant blood loss advantage with PSI,[7] whereas others have not.[3,8,13,16,21] The results of the authors' study also indicated that LOS after simultaneous bilateral TKA was no different when PSI was used, although a trend was found toward lower LOS with PSI. This finding of comparable LOS is similar to what other investigators have reported for unilateral TKA.[7,16] Conversely, Noble and colleagues[13] reported a small but significant reduction in LOS in a prospective randomized study of 15 PSI versus 14 non-PSI cruciate-retaining TKAs using the Visionaire system. LOS is an important variable influencing hospital costs after total joint arthroplasty, but other factors like patient comorbidities also influence it.[22]

Thromboembolism and Complications

Thromboembolism is another complication that can have significant effects after TKA. This process starts early during surgery with venous stasis caused by tourniquet use and vessel torsion with high flexion of the knee. Prolonged anesthetic and operative time have been shown to significantly increase the risk of thrombotic events,[23] and, therefore, the thromboembolic risk may be higher for simultaneous bilateral TKA. In 1 study, the rate of venous thromboembolism was 10.9% in simultaneous bilateral TKA versus 3.1% in unilateral procedures.[24] PE rates were also higher: 0.81 for unilateral TKA versus 1.44% for simultaneous bilateral procedures. Decreasing tourniquet time using PSI may lead to decreased thromboembolic events. In this study, no patient developed PE in either group, and the prevalence of venous thrombosis was comparable between groups. Both groups had similar rates of return to the operating room for MUA and 1 knee of 64 in the PSI group underwent reoperation for a deep hematoma (1.6%). The number of complications may be too small to make statistical comparisons between groups.

Limitations

The main weakness of the authors' study results from the limitations imposed by its retrospective, nonrandomized, nonblinded design. This introduced a selection bias because the surgeon and patients were allowed to choose the type of treatment. Another limitation is with respect to preoperative autologous blood donation. Autologous donation has been shown to cause preoperative anemia and increase the risk of perioperative

Table 3
Complications in study groups

Group	Deep Venous Thrombosis	Pulmonary Embolism	Reoperation	Manipulation Under Anesthesia (Stiffness)
PSI group	1	0	1 (Hematoma)	2
Non-PSI group	1	0	0	2

Table 4
Perioperative outcome measures patient-specific instrumentation versus non–patient-specific instrumentation unilateral total knee arthroplasty

Study	Alignment	Surgical Time	Blood Loss	Length of Stay	Other Measures	Study Design
Boonen et al,[7] 2013	Coronal alignment similar	Operative time 5 min shorter	Blood loss less by 100 mL	No differences	—	Prospective, double blind, randomized
Vundelinckx et al,[16] 2013	Coronal alignment similar	—	No differences	No differences	Similar pain and function outcome scores	Retrospective case control
Hamilton et al,[17] 2013	Coronal alignment similar	4 min longer PSI	—	—	Reduced trays	Prospective randomized
Chareancholvanich et al,[8] 2013	Coronal alignment similar	Operative time 5 min shorter	No differences	—	—	Prospective randomized
Noble et al,[13] 2012	Fewer outliers in coronal alignment	Shorter operative time	—	Decreased LOS	Smaller incision, fewer trays	Prospective randomized
Spencer et al,[21] 2009	2 Outliers in PSI group; none in other	14% Shorter tourniquet time	No differences	—	—	Initial experience; retrospective case control

transfusion. Although this is an important confounding variable, all patients were prescribed preoperative erythropoietin in conjunction with autologous blood donation, and both comparison groups received similar blood donation protocol. The short follow-up time of this study is another weakness, although this is primarily a study of perioperative outcome measures. Longer-term follow-up may elucidate other differences between cohorts. The study was also underpowered in detecting a significant difference in some of the outcome measures and complication rates.

SUMMARY

In conclusion, the authors found that the use of PSI resulted in reduction in tourniquet time as well as perioperative blood loss as measured by Hgb drop. Transfusion requirements, LOS, thromboembolism, and early complication rates were similar between groups. These procedures were performed by a high-volume knee surgeon and the results may not be applicable to lower-volume and less-experienced surgeons performing simultaneous bilateral TKA's. Further research in the forms of high-quality randomized trials and cost-benefit analyses may help in further consolidation of these findings.

REFERENCES

1. Iorio R, Robb WJ, Healy WL, et al. Orthopaedic surgeon workforce and volume assessment for total hip and knee replacement in the United States: preparing for an epidemic. J Bone Joint Surg Am 2008;90: 1598–605.
2. Duffy GP. Maximizing surgeon and hospital total knee arthroplasty volume using customized patient instrumentation and swing operating rooms. Am J Orthop 2011;40:5–8.
3. Lachiewicz PF, Henderson RA. Patient-specific instruments for total knee arthroplasty. J Am Acad Orthop Surg 2013;21:513–8.
4. Ng VY, DeClaire JH, Berend KR, et al. Improved accuracy of alignment with patient-specific positioning guides compared with manual instrumentation in TKA. Clin Orthop Relat Res 2012;470:99–107.
5. Barrack RL, Ruh EL, Williams BM, et al. Patient specific cutting blocks are currently of no proven value. J Bone Joint Surg Br 2012;94(11 Suppl A):95–9.
6. Nunley RM, Ellison BS, Ruh EL, et al. Are patient-specific cutting blocks cost-effective for total knee arthroplasty? Clin Orthop Relat Res 2012;470:889–94.
7. Boonen B, Schotanus MG, Kerens B, et al. Intra-operative results and radiological outcome of conventional and patient-specific surgery in total knee arthroplasty: a multicentre randomized controlled trial. Knee Surg Sports Traumatol Arthrosc 2013; 21:2206–12.
8. Choreanchulvanich K, Narkbunnam R, Pornrattanamaneewong C. A prospective randomised controlled study of patient-specific cutting guides compared with conventional instrumentation in total knee replacement. Bone Joint J 2013;95-B: 354–9.
9. Chen JY, Yeo SJ, Yew AK, et al. The radiological outcomes of patient-specific instrumentation versus conventional total knee arthroplasty. Knee Surg Sports Traumatol Arthrosc 2014;22(3):630–5.
10. Daniilidis K, Tibesku CO. A comparison of conventional and patient-specific instruments in total knee arthroplasty. Int Orthop 2014;38(3):503–8.
11. Lustig S, Scholes CJ, Oussedik SI, et al. Unsatisfactory accuracy as determined by computer navigation of visionaire patient-specific instrumentation for total knee arthroplasty. J Arthroplasty 2013;28:469–73.
12. Nam D, Maher PA, Rebolledo BJ, et al. Patient specific cutting guides versus an imageless, computer-assisted surgery system in total knee arthroplasty. Knee 2013;20(4):263–7.
13. Noble JW Jr, Moore CA, Liu N. The value of patient-matched instrumentation in total knee arthroplasty. J Arthroplasty 2012;27:153–5.
14. Nunley RM, Ellison BS, Zhu J, et al. Do patient-specific guides improve coronal alignment in total knee arthroplasty? Clin Orthop Relat Res 2012;470: 895–902.
15. Roh YW, Kim TW, Lee S, et al. Is TKA using patient-specific instruments comparable to conventional TKA? A randomized controlled study of one system. Clin Orthop Relat Res 2013;471(12):3988–95.
16. Vundelinckx BJ, Bruckers L, De Mulder K, et al. Functional and radiographic short-term outcome evaluation of the visionaire system, a patient-matched instrumentation system for total knee arthroplasty. J Arthroplasty 2013;28:964–70.
17. Hamilton WG, Parks NL, Saxena A. Patient-specific instrumentation does not shorten surgical time: a prospective randomized trial. J Arthroplasty 2013; 28:96–100.
18. Ethgen O, Bruyere O, Richy F, et al. Health-related quality of life in total hip and total knee arthroplasty: a qualitative and systematic review of literature. J Bone Joint Surg Am 2004;86(5):963–74.
19. Losina E, Walensky RP, Kessler CL, et al. Cost-effectiveness of total knee arthroplasty in the United States: Patient risk and hospital volume. Arch Intern Med 2009;169(12):1113–22.
20. Memtsoudis SG, Ma Y, González Della Valle A, et al. Perioperative outcomes after unilateral and bilateral total knee arthroplasty. Anesthesiology 2009;111(6): 1206–16.
21. Spencer BA, Mont MA, McGrath MS, et al. Initial experience with custom-fit total knee

replacement: intra-operative events and long-leg coronal alignment. Int Orthop 2009;33(6):1571–5.

22. Olthof M, Stevens M, Bulstra SK, et al. The association between comorbidity and length of hospital stay and costs in total hip arthroplasty patients: a systematic review. J Arthroplasty 2014;29(5): 1009–14.

23. Jaffer AK, Barsoum WK, Krebs V, et al. Duration of anesthesia and venous thromboembolism after hip and knee arthroplasty. Mayo Clin Proc 2005;80(6):732–8.

24. Levy YD, Hardwick ME, Copp SN, et al. Thrombosis incidence in unilateral vs simultaneous bilateral total knee arthroplasty with compression device prophylaxis. J Arthroplasty 2013;28(3):474–8.

Risk Assessment Tools Used to Predict Outcomes of Total Hip and Total Knee Arthroplasty

Joseph F. Konopka, MD, MSc*, Viktor J. Hansen, MD,
Harry E. Rubash, MD, Andrew A. Freiberg, MD

KEYWORDS

- Total knee arthroplasty • Total hip arthroplasty • Prediction tools • Nomograms

KEY POINTS

- Clinical tools have been developed to help predict outcomes in total joint arthroplasty (TJA) patients to aid efficient care delivery as demand for TJA increases.
- The Risk Assessment and Prediction Tool (RAPT) uses preoperative patient factors to predict patient need for an extended care facility after TJA. Our experience shows that length of stay and percentage of patients discharged home can be improved.
- The Predicting Location after Arthroplasty Nomogram (PLAN) is an alternative tool for predicting patient discharge needs.
- The Morbidity and Mortality Acute Predictor (arthro-MAP) uses patient characteristics and intraoperative factors to predict a patient's probability of significant postoperative complications.
- The Penn Arthroplasty Risk Score predicts a patient's need for postoperative intensive care unit monitoring.

INTRODUCTION

The demand for total knee arthroplasty (TKA) and total hip arthroplasty (THA) in the United States is growing rapidly. Kurtz and colleagues[1] projected the demand for primary THA to grow 174% to 572,000, and primary TKA to grow by 673% to 3.48 million procedures per year by 2030. Demand for THA and TKA revision procedures is likewise expected to experience a large increase in demand of 147% and 601% by 2030, respectively.[1] Hospital costs associated with total joint arthroplasty (TJA) were estimated at $30 billion in 2004, and are expected to increase as demand increases.[1]

TKA and THA are considered safe, long-term, cost-effective treatments for osteoarthritis[2–4] and it is therefore desirable that the growing demand be met. The predicted shortage of qualified arthroplasty surgeons in relation to the increasing demand represents an additional challenge.[5] The United States health care system's ability to meet the rapidly growing demand will be predicated on safe and efficient delivery.

The capacity to predict patient outcomes and needs preoperatively allows more efficient delivery of care, which increases the ability of joint replacement surgeons to meet this demand. Numerous clinical tools have been developed to predict a variety of TJA patient outcomes (**Table 1**). Such

The authors have nothing to disclose.
Department of Orthopedic Surgery, Yawkey Center for Outpatient Care, Massachusetts General Hospital, Suite 3B, 55 Fruit Street, Boston, MA 02114-2696, USA
* Corresponding author.
E-mail address: jkonopka@partners.org

Orthop Clin N Am 46 (2015) 351–362
http://dx.doi.org/10.1016/j.ocl.2015.02.004
0030-5898/15/$ – see front matter © 2015 Elsevier Inc. All rights reserved.

Table 1
Select risk assessment tools for total hip and knee arthroplasty patients

Study	Study Design	Patients (n)	Tool Name	Predicts	Variables Measured	Internal C-Statistic	Notes
Oldmeadow et al,[13] 2003	Prospective	520	RAPT	Postoperative rehabilitation need	(6) Age, gender, preoperative walking distance, gait aid, community support, home caregiver	0.75	Based on Australian population
Barsoum et al,[17] 2010	Retrospective	517	PLAN	Postoperative rehabilitation need	(17) Type of surgery, age, gender, BMI, comorbidities, preoperative ambulation status, predicted postoperative ambulation status, home environment variables (no. of steps, bedroom on first or second floor, bathroom on first or second floor), baseline caregiver assistance, home distance relative to the OR	0.867	Externally Validated
Wuerz et al,[21] 2014	Retrospective	3511	arthro-MAP	Postoperative complications	(8) Lowest intraoperative HR, EBL, preoperative BUN, procedure type, race, ASA score, comorbidities, presence of fracture	0.76	Awaiting external validation
Courtney et al,[30] 2014	Retrospective	1594	PARS	Postoperative ICU care need	(5) COPD, CHF, CAD, EBL >1000, intraoperative vasopressor use	0.822	7-point scale, with postoperative ICU care recommended if ≥3 points
Sabry et al,[34] 2014	Retrospective	314	Unnamed nomogram	Reinfection after 2-stage TKA revision for infection	(12) BMI, time from index surgery, duration of symptoms, number of previous surgeries, preoperative hemoglobin, soft tissue coverage required, prior infection in the same joint, previous 2-stage revision, type of organism, diabetes, immunocompromise, and heart disease	0.773	Not externally validated

Abbreviations: arthro-MAP, Morbidity and Mortality Acute Predictor; ASA, American Society of Anesthesiologists; BMI, body mass index; BUN, blood urea nitrogen; CAD, coronary artery disease; CHF, congestive heart failure; COPD, chronic obstructive pulmonary disease; EBL, estimated blood loss; HR, heart rate; ICU, intensive care unit; OR, operating room; PARS, Penn Arthroplasty Risk Score; PLAN, Predicting Location After Arthroplasty Nomogram; RAPT, Risk Assessment and Prediction Tool; TKA, total knee arthroplasty.

tools may facilitate efficient resource utilization by helping select better candidates for TJA, anticipating resource-intensive intensive care unit (ICU) monitoring, and encouraging timely planning for patient transition to an extended care facility. These tools may also allow for early planning of discharge and postoperative care, potentially reducing hospital length of stay (LOS). The financial savings associated with decreasing LOS have been documented extensively.[6,7] However, to meet the goal of increasing the productivity of joint replacement surgeons, tools must predict accurately meaningful clinical outcomes and be generalizable widely.

This article reviews recently proposed clinical tools for predicting risks and outcomes in THA and TKA patients. Our definition of a clinical tool includes "scoring systems, nomograms, and algorithms using preoperative or operative factors to predict outcomes or events in THA or TKA." Additionally, we share the Massachusetts General Hospital (MGH) experience with using the RAPT to predict the need for an extended care facility after TJA.

DEVELOPMENT OF CLINICAL TOOLS

Many recently proposed clinical tools have been developed using similar methodology, although the specific statistical methods may vary. First, an outcome of interest is identified. The outcome is often binary or categorical, such as postoperative discharge to an extended care facility. Next, based on a literature review and often expert opinion, a number of variables are identified that may be associated with the outcome of interest. These variables may include demographic data, comorbidities, preoperative function scores using validated instruments, or intraoperative factors such as estimated blood loss (EBL). These data, as well as the outcome of interest, are collected from a cohort of TJA patients, either retrospectively or prospectively. Univariate logistic regression is often first used to explore the association of each variable independently with the outcome of interest. Then, multiple logistic regression is used frequently to explore how well multiple variables explain the outcome of interest when used simultaneously. Variables are often considered for inclusion one at a time to assess whether they improve substantially how well the logistic regression model fits the observed data.

The predictive power of a model is typically evaluated using a C-statistic, which determines if the model predicts the outcome better than chance alone.[8] This is also known as the area under the receiver operating characteristic curve. Models are typically considered reasonable when the C-statistic is greater than 0.7 and strong when it exceeds 0.8.[8] The final multiple logistic regression model coefficients are subsequently converted into a more easily utilized clinical risk prediction tool or nomogram.[9]

Validation of the tool is essential before using it in clinical practice.[10,11] Most authors use "internal validation." Internal validation is based on the study's internal dataset, often using the C-statistic as a summary measurement. Internal validation may overestimate the performance of the tool.[12] External validation aims to address the accuracy of a model in patients from a different population with the same underlying disease. This step is particularly important for relatively small datasets.[10,11]

PREDICTION TOOLS FOR DISCHARGE TO EXTENDED CARE FACILITIES

Tools allowing the surgeon to predict the need for discharge to an extended care facility could potentially increase efficiency by reducing LOS in the acute setting. Such tools include the Risk Assessment and Prediction Tool (RAPT) and the Predicting Location after Arthroplasty Nomogram (PLAN).

The RAPT was developed in Australia in 2003 by Oldmeadow and colleagues[13] to predict whether TJA patients would require discharge to an extended care facility (Fig. 1). The system was developed using a cohort of patients that included primary THA and TKA patients, as well as revision and hemiarthroplasty patients. The tool uses 6 variables, including age, gender, preoperative ambulatory distance, use of a gait aid, community support, and presence of a home caregiver. The tool is scored on a 12-point scale, with fewer than 6 points predicting need for an extended care facility, and more than 9 points predicting discharge directly home. The tool correctly predicted discharge destination in 75% of the study sample.

In a follow-up study, the authors used the RAPT on 50 consecutive patients and found an increase in home discharges from 34% to 64%, an average 1.1-day decrease in LOS, and no increase in readmission rates.[14] Other authors have used the RAPT, demonstrating good predictive accuracy[15] and a low relative risk of complications in patients with a RAPT score of greater than 9.[16] In contrast with many of the other scores, the RAPT has been validated in multiple countries and continents with relatively similar results between the different institutions.

The PLAN was developed by the Cleveland Clinic to predict post-acute care needs as an

Risk Assessment and Prediction Tool (RAPT)

	Value	Score
1. What is your age group?	50-65 years	=2
	66-75 years	=1
	> 75 years	=0
2. Gender?	Male	=2
	Female	=1
3. How far, on average, can you walk?	Two blocks or more (+/- rests)	=2
(a block is 200 meters)	1-2 blocks (the shopping centre)	=1
	Housebound (most of the time)	=0
4. Which gait aid do you use?	None	=2
(more often than not)	Single point stick	=1
	Crutches/frame	=0
5. Do you use community supports?	None or one per week	=1
(home help, meals-on wheels, district nurse)	Two or more per week	=0
6. Will you live with someone who can care for	Yes	=3
you after your operation?	No	=0
	Your score (out of 12)	

KEY: Scores < 6 high risk...... prediction: discharge extended inpatient rehabilitation
Scores > 9 low risk.......... prediction: discharge directly home
Scores 6-9 medium risk ....prediction: additional intervention to discharge directly home

Patient's expectation of discharge destination is also a determinant. The prediction indicated by the score is discussed with the patient and a destination plan agreed to.

Patient's preference	Prediction (Score)	Agreed destination
....	....	....

Fig. 1. The Risk Assessment and Prediction Tool (RAPT) uses 6 preoperative variables to predict the need for discharge to an extended care facility. (*From* Oldmeadow LB, McBurney H, Robertson VJ. Predicting risk of extended inpatient rehabilitation after hip or knee arthroplasty. J Arthroplasty 2003;18:778; with permission.)

alternative to RAPT.[17] The authors were concerned that the RAPT may not be generalizable to US patients, particularly given that the average LOS in Australia at the time of the RAPT's development was 8.6 days. In contrast with the RAPT's 6 variables, the PLAN includes 17 preoperative variables (**Fig. 2**), and had a C-statistic of 0.867 with the study's internal sample of 517 patients. This compared favorably with only 0.565 for the RAPT. The authors also externally validated the tool using 150 patients from 3 different hospitals, with a C-statistic of 0.861. In the author's home institution, case managers prepare discharge to an extended care facility if the PLAN predicts less than a 50% chance of a direct discharge home. They reported a decrease in LOS of 0.9 days when using the PLAN.

Additional studies have identified key variables associated with a postoperative need for discharge to a rehabilitation facility, but did not propose a specific clinical tool. One study examined a large number of THA and TKA patients at 3 high-volume institutions, identifying age, American Society of Anesthesiologists (ASA) class, female gender, and Medicare insurance as predictors of the need for discharge to an extended care facility.[18] The authors also noted significant practice variation across the 3 sites. A smaller study compared 50

patients discharged to a skilled nursing facility (SNF) and 50 patients discharged to home, finding lower preoperative Timed Get up and Go scores (TUG), lower preoperative EuroQOL Five Dimensions Questionnaire (EQ-5D) scores. The study concluded that higher ASA, increased LOS, increased self-reported postoperative pain, and decreased physical therapy achievements are associated with discharge to a SNF.[19]

PREDICTION TOOLS FOR POSTOPERATIVE COMPLICATIONS

Predicting complications after surgery is a challenging problem. Cima and colleagues[20] recently compared the performance of the Agency for Healthcare Research and Quality Patient Safety Indictors (AHRQ-PSI) in predicting general and vascular surgery adverse events as identified by the American College of Surgeons National Surgical Quality Improvement Program (ACS-NSQIP). The AHRQ-PSI is a set of computer algorithms that predict potential adverse events based on procedure codes and secondary diagnoses. The ACS-NSQIP, on the other hand, uses manual review to apply risk-adjustment methodology to compare observed to expected outcomes in general and vascular surgery. The authors found that

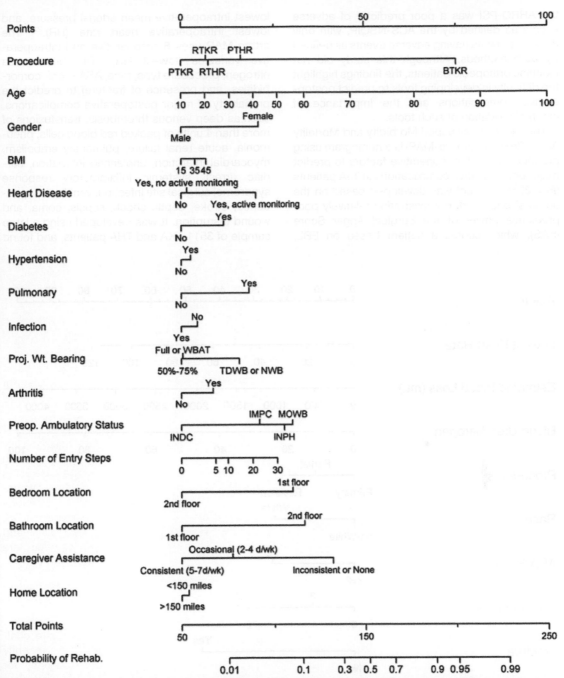

Fig. 2. The Predicting Location After Arthroplasty Nomogram (PLAN) uses 17 preoperative variables to predict the need for discharge to an extended care facility. To compute the predicted probability, a vertical line is drawn from the values of the individual variables to the scale for points in top. Then a vertical line from the total points is drawn to the corresponding probability. BMI, body mass index; BTKR, bilateral total knee replacement; IMPC, impaired community distances; INDC, independent community distances; INPH, impaired home distances; MOWB, minimal or wheelchair bound; NWB, non-weight bearing; PTHR, primary total hip replacement; PTKR, primary total knee replacement; RTHR, revision total hip replacement; RTKR, revision total knee replacement; TDWB, touch-down weight bearing; WBAT, weight bearing as tolerated. (*From* Barsoum WK, Murray TG, Klika AK, et al. Predicting patient discharge disposition after total joint arthroplasty in the United States. J Arthroplasty 2010;25:885–92; with permission.)

the AHRQ-PSI was a poor predictor of adverse events as defined by the ACS-NSQIP, with only 2.1% of patients having adverse events as defined by both methods. Although this study did not examine orthopedic patients, the findings highlight the difficulty in developing tools to predict postoperative complications and the importance of external validation of such tools.

The recently developed Morbidity and Mortality Acute Predictor (arthro-MAP) is a nomogram using preoperative and intraoperative factors to predict major postoperative complications in TJA patients (Fig. 3).[21] This tool was developed based on the authors' prior work demonstrating relatively poor predictive power of the Surgical Apgar Score (SAS), which scores a patient based on EBL,

lowest intraoperative mean arterial pressure, and lowest intraoperative heart rate (HR).[22] The arthro-MAP uses 8 preoperative and intraoperative variables (lowest HR, EBL, blood urea nitrogen, procedure type, race, ASA score, comorbidities, and presence of fracture) to predict the probability of major postoperative complications, such as deep venous thrombosis, transfusions of more than 4 units of packed red blood cells, pneumonia, acute renal failure, pulmonary embolism, myocardial infarction, unplanned intubation, cardiac arrest, systemic inflammatory response syndrome, surgical site infection, ventilator dependence, stroke, septic shock, sepsis, coma, and wound disruption. It was developed using a large sample of 3511 TKA and THA patients, and found

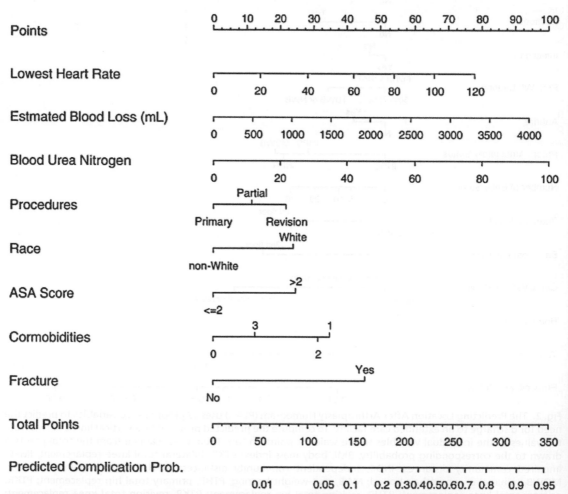

Fig. 3. The Morbidity and Mortality Acute Predictor (arthro-MAP) uses readily available preoperative and intraoperative factors to predict postoperative complications. To compute the predicted probability, a vertical line is drawn from the values of the individual variables to the scale for points in top. Then a vertical line from the total points is drawn to the corresponding probability. ASA, American Society of Anesthesiologists. (*From* Wuerz TH, Kent DM, Malchau H, et al. A nomogram to predict major complications after hip and knee arthroplasty. J Arthroplasty 2014;29:1460; with permission.)

to have a higher internal concordance index than the SAS (0.76 vs 0.61). The authors are currently validating the tool externally.

Other authors have developed statistical models predicting risk of postoperative complications without proposing a clinical tool. Hooper and colleagues[23] studied the relationship between ASA and 6-month mortality, 6-month Oxford Knee Scores (OKS), and prosthetic survival rates in a large cohort of patients from the New Zealand Joint Registry (22,600 THA and 18,434 TKA patients). ASA scores correlated strongly with 6-month mortality, with ASA 1 THA patients having 0.12% mortality at 6 months and ASA 4 patients undergoing THA having 10.06% mortality at 6 months. Although ASA scores correlated with OKS scores at 6 months, the authors measured only absolute OKS scores, not the change in OKS scores. Higher ASA scores were likewise predictive of revision THA within 2 years; however, it was not predictive of revision TKA.

Marin and colleagues[24] examined the ability of preoperative nutrition laboratory tests to predict wound healing in arthroplasty patients. The small sample size of only 46 patients limited development of a clinical tool. However, they found that preoperative lymphocyte levels of less than 1500 were associated with a 3-fold greater risk of wound complications, including drainage or some degree of wound dehiscence. Although not a tool, this information is often routinely obtained in preoperative laboratory tests and may increase the surgeon's index of suspicion.

Inneh and colleagues[25] retrospectively reviewed 5134 THA and TKA patients and found that an ASA of greater than 2, advanced age, prolonged operating time, and preexisting genitourinary, circulatory, respiratory, and mental health conditions were predictive of orthopedic and nonorthopedic complications, including readmission within 30 days. Voskuijl and colleagues[26] found that the Charlson Comorbidity Index (CCI) score was predictive of readmission rates and transfusion rates in arthroplasty, but that it had poor explanatory power if used in isolation. Pavesi and colleagues[27] developed a model to predict the need for postoperative transfusion in THA. This model uses patient age, gender, and preoperative hemoglobin level to predict if the postoperative hemoglobin level is expected to decrease to below 10.

PREDICTION TOOLS FOR POSTOPERATIVE INTENSIVE CARE UNIT MONITORING

Unplanned ICU admissions are associated with high patient mortality.[28] Furthermore, ICU costs account for approximately 1 of every 3 health care

dollars spent.[29] The ability to identify patients at risk for ICU intervention, therefore, has the potential to both improve outcomes and reduce costs.

The Penn Arthroplasty Risk Score (PARS) was developed to help identify arthroplasty patients who would require ICU intervention postoperatively, thereby enhancing postoperative ICU triage and preventing unplanned ICU admissions (**Fig. 4**).[30] This tool uses 5 variables including chronic obstructive pulmonary disease (1 point), congestive heart failure (1 point), coronary artery disease (1 point), EBL greater than 1000 mL (2 points), and intraoperative vasopressin use (2 points). Using this model, 4 and 7 points indicated a 55.4% and 83.4% probability of needing ICU intervention, respectively. The authors noted a C-statistic of 0.822 using their internal cohort of 1594 TKA and THA patients. At the authors' institution, patients are sent to the ICU for postoperative monitoring if the patient has a PARS score of 3 or higher.

Kamath and colleagues[31] identified variables that are predictive for unplanned ICU admissions. In a retrospective study of 1259 THA patients, they identified age greater than 75 years, BMI greater than 35 kg/m^2, creatinine clearance less than 60 mL/min, revision surgery, and previous myocardial infarction as independent risk factors for an unplanned ICU admission. Although not a clinical tool, the authors currently plan an ICU admission if the patient has several of these characteristics.

PREDICTION TOOLS FOR LENGTH OF STAY

We did not identify a clinical tool that was highly predictive of postoperative LOS in a United States population. Ong and colleagues[32] developed a 13-variable nomogram to predict LOS in TKA and unicompartmental knee arthroplasty patients in Singapore; however, this model explained only 32% of the variation in LOS. Additionally, given the high average LOS of 5 days at the authors' institution, this may not be easily generalizable to a United States population. Styron and colleagues[7] used data from the Health Care Utilization Project to examine a very large number of discharges (322,894 THA and 193,553 TKA) for the effects of both patient and provider characteristics on LOS. The authors found that both patient and provider characteristics mattered. The variables that had the greatest effect were a high Charlson Comorbidity Index (CCI), low surgeon volume, and low hospital volume. This study highlights generalizability issues for applying tools created in high-volume centers to low-volume hospitals and surgeons, particularly when predicting LOS.

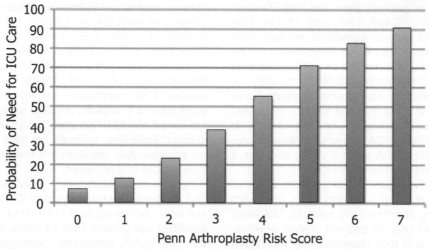

Penn Arthroplasty Risk Score	Points
Chronic Obstructive Pulmonary Disease	1
Congestive Heart Failure	1
Coronary Artery Disease	1
EBL > 1000	2
Intraoperative Vasopressors	2
TOTAL	7

Fig. 4. The Penn Arthroplasty Risk Score (PARS) uses 5 preoperative and intraoperative variables to predict the risk of an ICU intervention. The authors admit patients to the ICU postoperative if their PARS score is 3 or greater. EBL, estimated blood loss. (*From* Courtney PM, Whitaker CM, Gutsche JT, et al. Predictors of the need for critical care after total joint arthroplasty: an update of our institutional risk stratification model. J Arthroplasty 2014;29:1350–4; with permission.)

PREDICTION TOOLS FOR SUCCESSFUL TREATMENT OF PROSTHETIC JOINT INFECTIONS

Buller and colleagues[33] created a 14-variable nomogram predicting the risk of reinfection after incision and drainage (I&D) as well as liner exchange in TKA and THA. The study was based on 309 retrospective patients and had a concordance index of 0.645. To our knowledge, the nomogram has not been validated externally. Although the concordance index is relatively low, it offers a more sophisticated approach to the choice to perform an I&D and liner exchange over the traditional method of selection based on duration of symptoms of less than 4 weeks.

Sabry and colleagues[34] designed a 12-point nomogram to predict the risk of reinfection after a 2-stage TKA revision for infection (**Fig. 5**). This nomogram was based on 314 two-stage revisions. It had a C-statistic of 0.773. Although promising, it has not been validated externally. Kubista and colleagues[35] had investigated previously risk factors that were predictive of reinfection after a 2-stage revision, but had not proposed a clinical tool.

PREDICTION TOOLS FOR PATIENT FUNCTIONAL OUTCOMES

The Risk Score Points System was developed to predict long-term benefit after THA.[36] The system uses preoperative Short Form (SF)-36 scores, gender, age, radiographic grade of hip osteoarthritis, history of prior hip injury, and the number of painful joints to predict a greater than 30-point improvement in SF-36 physical function scores at 8 years postoperatively. It has not been validated externally and was based on a retrospective study of 282 patients in England. Nonetheless, it demonstrated good predictive power internally, with a C-statistic of 0.74.

Other authors have investigated tools and predictive factors for a variety of functional outcomes at 6 months postoperatively. Bade and colleagues[37] created a regression model using preoperative TKA physical therapy tests, demonstrating that preoperative performance on Timed Up and Go tests (TUG), 6-minute walk distance, and stair climbing tests were highly predictive of improvements in these measures at 6 months postoperatively. However, this study is limited by

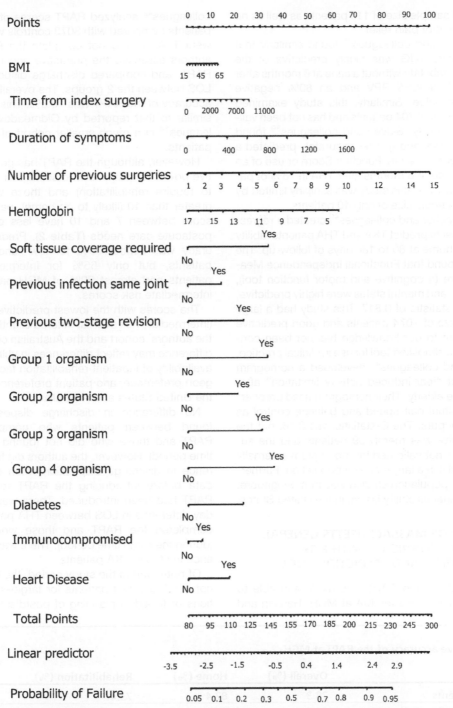

Fig. 5. A 12-point nomogram to predict the chance of reinfection after a 2-stage total knee arthroplasty revision for infection. To compute the predicted probability, a vertical line is drawn from the values of the individual variables to the scale for points in top. Then a vertical line from the total points is drawn to the corresponding probability. BMI, body mass index. (*From* Sabry FY, Buller L, Ahmed S, et al. Preoperative prediction of failure following two-stage revision for knee prosthetic joint infections. J Arthroplasty 2014;29:120; with permission.)

the small sample size of 119 patients as well as no assessment of pain relief.

Nankaku and colleagues[38] found similarly that preoperative TUG was highly predictive of the ability to ambulate without a cane at 6 months after THA, with a 92% PPV and an 80% negative predictive value. Similarly, this study examined a small group of 204 patients and has not been validated externally. Slaven and colleagues[39] found that BMI, age, and gender accurately predicted a poor Lower Extremity Function Score or use of an assist device at 6 months after THA in 78% of patients. However, this study was similarly limited by its small sample size of only 40 patients.

Ottenbacher and colleagues[40] created a regression model to predict TKA and THA patients' ability to live at home at 80 to 180 days of follow-up. The authors found that Functional Independence Measure score (a cognitive and motor function tool), LOS, age, and marital status were highly predictive, with a C-statistic of 0.817. This study had a large sample size of 7074 patients and good predictive power, but to our knowledge has not been converted to a simplified tool for use in clinical practice.

Pua and colleagues[41] developed a nomogram to predict "fear-induced activity limitation" after TKA in the elderly. Their nomogram used preoperative habitual gait speed and balance control as the only inputs. The C-statistic was 0.76, but the sample size was merely 39 patients and the authors have not validated this nomogram externally or studied it in a larger patient population. Furthermore, the population studied was from Singapore, raising generalizability issues in the United States.

RESULTS OF MASSACHUSETTS GENERAL HOSPITAL EXPERIENCE WITH RISK ASSESSMENT AND PREDICTION TOOL

In June 2006, the RAPT was made available to patients scheduled for TJA at MGH. Hansen and colleagues[42] analyzed RAPT scores of 3213 TJA patients compared with 3073 controls who underwent TJA but did not complete the RAPT. The authors assessed the predictive accuracy of the RAPT, and compared discharge disposition and LOS between the 2 groups. The overall predictive accuracy of the RAPT was 78.3%. This value was similar to that reported by Oldmeadow and colleagues[14] in a much smaller cohort of Australian patients.

However, although the RAPT has good predictive power for patients who score 6 or less (likely to require rehabilitation) and those who score greater than 10 (likely to go home), patients who score between 7 and 10 have less predictable postacute care needs (**Table 2**). Predictive accuracy was almost 90% for low- and high-risk patients, but only 65% for intermediate risk patients and almost 50% of MGH patients had intermediate risk scores.

The scores with the lowest predictive accuracy (intermediate risk scores) differed slightly between the authors' cohort and the Australian cohort. This difference may reflect differences in utilization and availability of inpatient rehabilitation facilities, surgeon preference, and patient preference between the United States and Australia.

No difference in discharge disposition was found between patients who completed the RAPT and those who did not (during the same time period). However, the authors did find a difference in discharge disposition when comparing data before introducing the RAPT to after the RAPT had been introduced. There was an 0.73-day difference in LOS between THA patients who completed the RAPT and those who did not (during the same time period). There was no difference in LOS in TKA patients.

Of note, during the study period, the RAPT was not used to select patients for targeted interventions or to aid in planning of postdischarge care

Table 2				
Predictive accuracy of the RAPT at MGH				
Cohort	Overall (%)	Home (%)	Rehabilitation (%)	P Value
All patients	78.3	82.4	73.4	<.0001
THA	79.6	91.1	63.0	<.0001
TKA	77.4	83.3	71.3	<.0001
High risk (0–6)	89.4	0.0	100.0	<.0001
Intermediate risk (7–10)	65.2	100.0	0.0	<.0001
Low risk (11–12)	89.5	100.0	0.0	<.0001

Abbreviations: MGH, Massachusetts General Hospital; RAPT, Risk Assessment and Prediction Tool; THA, total hip arthroplasty; TKA, total knee arthroplasty.

Adapted from Hansen VJ, Gromov K, Lebrun LM, et al. Risk assessment tools used to predict outcomes of total hip and total knee arthroplasty. Clin Orthop Relat Res 2015;473(2):597–601; with permission.

during the study period. The authors purposely excluded data for 2012 and 2013, because during those years the RAPT was actually used for these purposes and they felt that interventions based on the RAPT would alter the predictive accuracy of the tool by increasing it falsely. Although there was no difference in discharge disposition and only a small difference in LOS between patients who completed the RAPT and those who did not, the authors concluded that LOS and percentage of patients that are discharge home can be improved when using the RAPT to make clinical decisions and plan postoperative care.

SUMMARY

A variety of clinical tools have been developed over the last decade to predict a variety of outcomes in TJA patients. Our own experience using RAPT at MGH has demonstrated good predictive accuracy and, although it has not decreased LOS unequivocally, it assists with identification of patients for targeted interventions to facilitate discharge home. Although several tools have demonstrated promising predictive power with internal validation, few tools have been validated externally. Additional studies are needed to validate externally promising tools such as the arthro-MAP and PARS.

REFERENCES

1. Kurtz S, Ong K, Lau E, et al. Projections of primary and revision hip and knee arthroplasty in the United States from 2005 to 2030. J Bone Joint Surg Am 2007;89:780–5.
2. Losina E, Walensky RP, Kessler CL, et al. Cost-effectiveness of total knee arthroplasty in the United States: patient risk and hospital volume. Arch Intern Med 2009;169:1113–21 [discussion: 1121–2].
3. Lavernia CJ, Guzman JF, Gachupin-Garcia A. Cost effectiveness and quality of life in knee arthroplasty. Clin Orthop Relat Res 1997;(345):134–9.
4. Ethgen O, Bruyere O, Richy F, et al. Health-related quality of life in total hip and total knee arthroplasty. A qualitative and systematic review of the literature. J Bone Joint Surg Am 2004;86-A:963–74.
5. Fehring TK, Odum SM, Troyer JL, et al. Joint replacement access in 2016: a supply side crisis. J Arthroplasty 2010;25:1175–81.
6. Healy WL, Iorio R, Richards JA, et al. Opportunities for control of hospital costs for total joint arthroplasty after initial cost containment. J Arthroplasty 1998;13:504–7.
7. Styron JF, Koroukian SM, Klika AK, et al. Patient vs provider characteristics impacting hospital lengths of stay after total knee or hip arthroplasty. J Arthroplasty 2011;26:1418–26.e1–2.
8. Hosmer DW. Applied logistic regression. 2nd edition. New York: John Wiley & Sons; 2000.
9. van Staa TP, Geusens P, Kanis JA, et al. A simple clinical score for estimating the long-term risk of fracture in post-menopausal women. QJM 2006;99:673–82.
10. Bleeker SE, Moll HA, Steyerberg EW, et al. External validation is necessary in prediction research: a clinical example. J Clin Epidemiol 2003;56:826–32.
11. Steyerberg EW, Bleeker SE, Moll HA, et al. Internal and external validation of predictive models: a simulation study of bias and precision in small samples. J Clin Epidemiol 2003;56:441–7.
12. Steyerberg EW, Harrell FE Jr, Borsboom GJ, et al. Internal validation of predictive models: efficiency of some procedures for logistic regression analysis. J Clin Epidemiol 2001;54:774–81.
13. Oldmeadow LB, McBurney H, Robertson VJ. Predicting risk of extended inpatient rehabilitation after hip or knee arthroplasty. J Arthroplasty 2003;18:775–9.
14. Oldmeadow LB, McBurney H, Robertson VJ, et al. Targeted postoperative care improves discharge outcome after hip or knee arthroplasty. Arch Phys Med Rehabil 2004;85:1424–7.
15. Tan C, Loo G, Pua YH, et al. Predicting discharge outcomes after total knee replacement using the Risk Assessment and Predictor Tool. Physiotherapy 2014;100:176–81.
16. Dauty M, Schmitt X, Menu P, et al. Using the Risk Assessment and Predictor Tool (RAPT) for patients after total knee replacement surgery. Ann Phys Rehabil Med 2012;55:4–15.
17. Barsoum WK, Murray TG, Klika AK, et al. Predicting patient discharge disposition after total joint arthroplasty in the United States. J Arthroplasty 2010;25:885–92.
18. Bozic KJ, Wagie A, Naessens JM, et al. Predictors of discharge to an inpatient extended care facility after total hip or knee arthroplasty. J Arthroplasty 2006;21:151–6.
19. Sharareh B, Le NB, Hoang MT, et al. Factors determining discharge destination for patients undergoing total joint arthroplasty. J Arthroplasty 2014;29:1355–8.e1.
20. Cima RR, Lackore KA, Nehring SA, et al. How best to measure surgical quality? Comparison of the Agency for Healthcare Research and Quality Patient Safety Indicators (AHRQ-PSI) and the American College of Surgeons National Surgical Quality Improvement Program (ACS-NSQIP) postoperative adverse events at a single institution. Surgery 2011;150:943–9.
21. Wuerz TH, Kent DM, Malchau H, et al. A nomogram to predict major complications after hip and knee arthroplasty. J Arthroplasty 2014;29:1457–62.
22. Wuerz TH, Regenbogen SE, Ehrenfeld JM, et al. The Surgical Apgar Score in hip and knee arthroplasty. Clin Orthop Relat Res 2011;469:1119–26.

23. Hooper GJ, Rothwell AG, Hooper NM, et al. The relationship between the American Society Of Anesthesiologists physical rating and outcome following total hip and knee arthroplasty: an analysis of the New Zealand Joint Registry. J Bone Joint Surg Am 2012;94:1065–70.

24. Marin LA, Salido JA, Lopez A, et al. Preoperative nutritional evaluation as a prognostic tool for wound healing. Acta Orthop Scand 2002;73:2–5.

25. Inneh IA, Lewis CG, Schutzer SF. Focused risk analysis: regression model based on 5,314 total hip and knee arthroplasty patients from a single institution. J Arthroplasty 2014;29(10):2031–5.

26. Voskuijl T, Hageman M, Ring D. Higher Charlson Comorbidity Index scores are associated with readmission after orthopaedic surgery. Clin Orthop Relat Res 2014;472:1638–44.

27. Pavesi M, Inghilleri G, Albano G, et al. A predictive model to reduce allogenic transfusions in primary total hip arthroplasty. Transfus Apher Sci 2011;45:265–8.

28. Liu V, Kipnis P, Rizk NW, et al. Adverse outcomes associated with delayed intensive care unit transfers in an integrated healthcare system. J Hosp Med 2012;7:224–30.

29. Shorr AF. An update on cost-effectiveness analysis in critical care. Curr Opin Crit Care 2002;8:337–43.

30. Courtney PM, Whitaker CM, Gutsche JT, et al. Predictors of the need for critical care after total joint arthroplasty: an update of our institutional risk stratification model. J Arthroplasty 2014;29:1350–4.

31. Kamath AF, McAuliffe CL, Gutsche JT, et al. Intensive care monitoring after total joint replacement. Bone Joint J 2013;95-B:74–6.

32. Ong PH, Pua YH. A prediction model for length of stay after total and unicompartmental knee replacement. Bone Joint J 2013;95-B:1490–6.

33. Buller LT, Sabry FY, Easton RW, et al. The preoperative prediction of success following irrigation and debridement with polyethylene exchange for hip and knee prosthetic joint infections. J Arthroplasty 2012;27:857–64.e1–4.

34. Sabry FY, Buller L, Ahmed S, et al. Preoperative prediction of failure following two-stage revision for knee prosthetic joint infections. J Arthroplasty 2014;29:115–21.

35. Kubista B, Hartzler RU, Wood CM, et al. Reinfection after two-stage revision for periprosthetic infection of total knee arthroplasty. Int Orthop 2012;36:65–71.

36. Judge A, Javaid MK, Arden NK, et al. Clinical tool to identify patients who are most likely to achieve long-term improvement in physical function after total hip arthroplasty. Arthritis Care Res 2012;64:881–9.

37. Bade MJ, Wolfe P, Zeni JA, et al. Predicting poor physical performance after total knee arthroplasty. J Orthop Res 2012;30:1805–10.

38. Nankaku M, Tsuboyama T, Akiyama H, et al. Preoperative prediction of ambulatory status at 6 months after total hip arthroplasty. Phys Ther 2013;93:88–93.

39. Slaven EJ. Prediction of functional outcome at six months following total hip arthroplasty. Phys Ther 2012;92:1386–94.

40. Ottenbacher KJ, Smith PM, Illig SB, et al. Prediction of follow-up living setting in patients with lower limb joint replacement. Am J Phys Med Rehabil 2002;81:471–7.

41. Pua YH, Ong PH, Lee AY, et al. Preliminary prediction model for fear-induced activity limitation after total knee arthroplasty in people 60 years and older: prospective cohort study. Arch Phys Med Rehabil 2013;94(3):503–9.

42. Hansen VJ, Gromov K, Lebrun LM, et al. Does the risk assessment and prediction tool predict discharge disposition after joint replacement? Clin Orthop Relat Res 2015;473(2):597–601.

Trauma

Preface

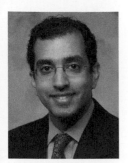

Saqib Rehman, MD
Editor

Tibial plateau fractures present with a spectrum of injury from simple unicondylar, partial articular fractures with mild soft tissue injury to complex bicondylar patterns with depression, meniscal injury, and soft tissue compromise. Having a thorough understanding of the pitfalls in the management of these injuries is important to stay out of trouble and achieve good outcomes. Not only is it important to be facile with the surgical techniques of treating these injuries but also it is equally important to understand the indications for applying different surgical approaches and fixation methods, and the appropriate timing of surgical intervention. Drs Yoon, Liporace, and Egol present a thorough review of the definitive treatment of tibial plateau fractures that will be helpful for those surgeons who see these injuries in their practice. I hope you enjoy this article and this issue of the *Orthopedic Clinics of North America*.

Saqib Rehman, MD
Department of Orthopaedic Surgery
Temple University Hospital
3401 North Broad Street
Philadelphia, PA 19140, USA

E-mail address:
Saqib.rehman@tuhs.temple.edu

Orthop Clin N Am 46 (2015) xv
http://dx.doi.org/10.1016/j.ocl.2015.03.002
0030-5898/15/$ – see front matter © 2015 Published by Elsevier Inc.

Definitive Fixation of Tibial Plateau Fractures

Richard S. Yoon, MD, Frank A. Liporace, MD, Kenneth A. Egol, MD*

KEYWORDS

• Tibial plateau fracture • Operative management • Internal fixation • Outcomes

KEY POINTS

• Always evaluate mechanism of injury and associated energy.
• Rule out neurovascular injury, and have a low threshold and suspicion for compartment syndrome.
• Be aware of soft tissue condition—implementing a staged protocol with external fixator can allow for a more ideal surgical environment.
• Obtain advanced imaging (CT) before definitive treatment to understand the fracture personality.
• Apply surgical approach and fixation strategy to personality of each fracture.
• Never compromise exposure for cosmesis.
• Multiple surgical approaches, even in a staged fashion, may be necessary.

INTRODUCTION

In regards to operative fixation of tibial plateau fractures, classical Arbeitsgemeinschaft für Osteosynthesefragen (AO) teaching emphasized the importance of anatomic articular restoration and stable fixation to allow for early range of knee motion.[1,2] However, early results, secondary to excessive soft tissue stripping and overly rigid fixation, led to undesirable high nonunion rates and failure.[3] However, the paradigm and strategy in the operative treatment of tibial plateau fractures has evolved dramatically in recent years. Nuances in anatomic approaches, advances in implant technology, and an improved respect and understanding for surgical technique and the surrounding soft tissue envelope have allowed for improved short- and long-term results.[4–6]

Tibial plateau fractures occur in all age groups, but generally have a bimodal distribution within a given population occurring in young adults as a result of high-energy trauma, and in the elderly as a result of low-energy injuries. There is a spectrum of injury, with the severity of each fracture dependent on the mechanism of injury, the associated energy, and the quality of the host bone. However, despite the variety in which these fracture patterns can occur, the goals and principles remain the same: restoration of the articular surface and maintenance of the mechanical axis. However, depending on the specific type of fracture pattern, implementing the proper planning, surgical technique, and management can help to maximize clinical outcomes, while avoiding complications.

This article helps the reader achieve those goals by summarizing the pertinent principles, strategies, and techniques for some of the most commonly presenting tibial plateau fractures. This is achieved via a case-based platform in hopes of providing a more individualized approach that can be readily implemented across a wide audience.

The authors have nothing to disclose.
Division of Orthopaedic Trauma, Department of Orthopaedic Surgery, NYU Hospital for Joint Diseases, NYU langone medical center, 301 East 17th Street, Suite 1402, New York, NY 10003, USA
* Corresponding author.
E-mail address: Kenneth.egol@nyumc.org

Orthop Clin N Am 46 (2015) 363–375
http://dx.doi.org/10.1016/j.ocl.2015.02.005
0030-5898/15/$ – see front matter © 2015 Elsevier Inc. All rights reserved.

orthopedic.theclinics.com

IMPORTANT CONSIDERATIONS BEFORE SURGERY

Arguably, once appropriately indicated, the most important stage of treating tibial plateau fractures occurs before entering the operating room. Preoperative planning, which includes evaluation and decision for surgery, diagnostic and advanced imaging, along with timing and formulation of a surgical plan not only help to achieve a desired clinical result, but aid the surgeon in execution of the procedure.

Surgical planning begins with the initial evaluation and interview. Assessing the mechanism and energy of the sustained injury along with a thorough medical history can provide a general outline of the underlying fracture pattern, and the fixation and management strategy that may ultimately be required. For example, the injury pattern for a 24-year-old man who presents after a high-energy motorcycle crash differs from that of a 78-year-old woman who sustained a low-energy valgus load to the knee while grocery shopping. Coinciding with obtaining a thorough history is a complete physical examination. Neurovascular assessment, including measuring ankle-brachial indices (ABI), should be performed if there is any suspicion for vascular compromise that could be a hard sign, such as diminished pulses, or a soft sign, such as fracture pattern. Furthermore, initial assessment of the surrounding soft tissue envelope can indicate not only the severity of the fracture, but may also provide an approximate timeline to definitive fixation. Ligamentous assessment, although important in high-energy plateau fracture-dislocations, may be difficult to assess on initial presentation because of pain and swelling.

No matter how thorough a history and physical examination is performed, diagnosis and operative planning cannot start without obtaining appropriate imaging. Anteroposterior (AP), lateral, and oblique views should be initially obtained. Tibial plateau views, directed in line with the anatomic 10-degree slope of the tibia, can also be helpful, although with the advent of more advanced imaging modalities (ie, computed tomography [CT]), it is rarely obtained. Initial diagnosis via plain radiographs, combined with knowing the mechanism and energy of the injury, is of paramount importance because it dictates the next stage in management. For low-energy injuries with relatively simple fracture patterns, immobilization with plaster or a knee immobilizer and an immediate CT should be the next step. However, for higher-energy injuries with associated complex fracture patterns and significant soft tissue damage, the decision to temporarily stabilize with external fixation is made.

Ideally, classification systems should not only have high agreement between observers, but should also provide consistent reliable agreement on treatment and prognosis. However, most classification systems fall short on each of those ideals, and tibial plateau fractures are no different. Most commonly, the Schatzker, the Moore, and the AO/Orthopaedic Trauma Association (OTA) classifications have been used.[3,7,8] Using radiographs alone, Maripuri and colleagues[9] reported moderate agreement between observers, the best agreement exhibited with the Schatzker classification. Adding CT, however, improves observer agreement from moderate to good.[10] If observers are provided with three-dimensional reconstructions, agreement improves to excellent for the Schatzker classification.[11]

The role of CT in regards to operative planning cannot be understated. Close analysis of CT reconstructions in the axial, coronal, and sagittal planes can offer key insight into the degree of injury by revealing entrance and exiting locations of major fracture lines, extent and location of column involvement and articular depression, degree of comminution, and any distal extension into the meta-diaphyseal junction.

In turn, understanding these key components of any tibial plateau fracture helps plan for specific approaches and implant and bone void filler selection. Additionally, for those patterns with increasing levels of articular depression and higher-energy fracture patterns, meniscal injury and/or associated ligamentous injury can be expected.[12–14]

DEFINITIVE FIXATION SHOULD FOLLOW SOFT TISSUE RESOLUTION

Tibial plateau fractures can often present with significant soft tissue injury not amenable to acute, definitive fixation. Ignoring soft tissue quality can lead to high rates of infection and complications, especially during the first 7 days after injury.[15–18] Complications arise from the underlying inflammatory cascade that leads to venous congestion, hypoxia, and subsequent necrosis creating the least ideal operative environment.[19,20]

Drawing from the staged protocol used for pilon fracture management, the same can be applied to tibial plateau fractures to allow for optimum soft tissue status before definitive fixation.[21,22] Egol and colleagues,[22] using spanning external fixation for high-energy proximal tibial fractures, reported low wound complication rates. With minimal soft tissue complications, the group recommended staged fixation for all high-energy fractures of the proximal tibia. Temporary (or in some cases, definitive) external fixation not only provides skeletal stabilization to maintain length, alignment, and rotation, but also allows for easy access for wound and blister management (**Fig. 1**).

Finally, although still controversial, one must be cognizant of pin-site placement in regards to future plate placement. Although classic teaching recommends placement of pin-sites outside of the zone of future plate placement, there is a paucity of literature to suggest if it truly holds an increased infection rate.[23] Recent studies, in an effort to provide objective data to find an answer, reported conflicting results.[24,25] In a small cohort comparison study, Laible and colleagues[24] did not find an increased infection rate in tibial plateau fractures fixed with plates that overlapped with pin-sites. Shah and colleagues[25] found the opposite, finding an increased infection rate with plate, pin-site overlap. However, the authors had a more heterogeneous study cohort, including both tibial plafond and plateau fractures.[25] While we await larger studies for a definitive answer based on objective data, we recommend trying to place pin-sites outside of the zone of fixation. However, that goal should not outweigh achieving stability, length, and alignment.

DEFINITIVE FIXATION: CASE-BASED STRATEGIES AND TECHNIQUES

Goals for definitive fixation for tibial plateau fractures revolve around implementing basic principles to achieve good outcomes (**Box 1**). Certain techniques and strategies can be implemented for specific fracture patterns to achieve desired goals. The following scenarios represent some of the more commonly presenting fracture patterns, from the simple to the complex, with the specific

---

> **Box 1**
> **Principles of definitive fixation for tibial plateau fractures**
>
> 1. Restoration of articular surface, and mechanical axis alignment
>   - Do not forget about mechanical alignment
> 2. Balanced fixation: use appropriate hardware
>   - Match fixation strategy to the personality of the fracture pattern
>   - Raft subchondral bone either with screws alone or via plate
>   - No need to fill every hole with locking screws, use nonlocking where appropriate
>   - Buttress plating is your workhorse
> 3. Always remember to RESPECT THE SOFT TISSUES
>   - Only operate when soft tissues are ready (ie, skin wrinkling, minimal blisters)
>   - Use percutaneous and minimally invasive when appropriate
>   - However, expose as much as needed (never sacrifice to be minimally invasive)

---

techniques and strategies that can be applied to maximize outcomes.

Scenario 1: Simple Split Fractures

For simple split fracture patterns, Koval and colleagues[26] showed that excellent results could be achieved with indirect reduction techniques and percutaneous fixation. This has become a reproducible, reliable technique, but in the correct patient with the correct fracture pattern. Either tibial plateau views or a CT should be obtained to rule out any significant joint depression. If slight joint

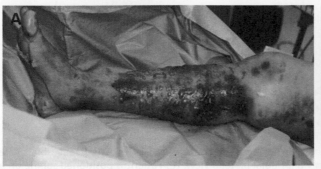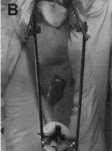

Fig. 1. Tibial plateau fractures often present with significant soft tissue injury that requires external stabilization. (*A*) A 37-year-old man with high-energy tibial plateau fracture after motorcycle crash with significant soft tissue injury. (*B*) A 46-year-old man after high-energy fall, with significant blistering with underlying tibial plateau fracture.

depression exists along with the split, percutaneous techniques and methods of elevating the joint line have also been developed.[27,28] However, we prefer to reserve the truly percutaneous and indirect reduction techniques for the pure split fractures. For split-depression fracture patterns, we typically formally open the fracture to visualize and assess and confirm anatomic articular reduction (Scenario 2).

Here we illustrate a 57-year-old woman who was struck by a bicyclist. Radiographs revealed an isolated split tibial plateau fracture (**Fig. 2**A), which we confirmed to be without depression via tibial plateau view (see **Fig. 2**B). Patient positioning and setup is the same setup used for all tibial plateau fractures. The patients should be supine on a radiolucent table, with a bump placed under the ischial tuberosity on the ipsilateral side along with fluoroscopic imaging placed on the contralateral side; placing the affected limb on a radiolucent knee triangle also helps to eliminate the uninjured leg, allowing for easily obtained images (see **Fig. 2**C).

Before reduction, it is important to replicate the tibial plateau view. Replicating the view and eliminating the posterior slope allows for a better assessment of the articular surface and therefore, the reduction obtained. This is another reason why we often obtain a tibial plateau view, because we use it intraoperatively as a comparison to our fluoroscopic images. Following confirmation of reduction, a large pointed reduction clamp can be used to obtain provisional reduction (see **Fig. 2**D). Care must be taken to avoid undesired pressure on the skin over the anterior aspect of the tibia. Finally, the reduction can be held provisionally with wire fixation, which can subsequently be replaced with partially threaded cannulated screws. Our

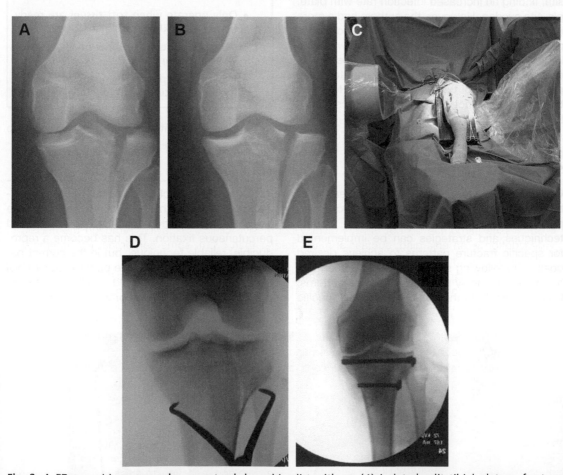

Fig. 2. A 57-year-old woman who was struck by a bicyclist with an (*A*) isolated split tibial plateau fracture, confirmed to be without depression via (*B*) tibial plateau view. (*C*) Patient is positioned supine on a radiolucent table, with a bump placed under the ischial tuberosity on the ipsilateral side on a radiolucent triangle; fluoroscopic imaging comes in from the contralateral side. (*D*) Reduction is obtained with a large pointed reduction clamp on the tibial plateau view and after provisional fixation with wires, (*E*) partially threaded cannulated screws and washers complete definitive fixation.

preference is to place a minimum of two screws along the subchondral surface and a third screw at the distal apex of the fracture (see **Fig. 2**E). We also use washers to increase the surface area, achieving more compression, and also it is important to sequentially tighten each screw to achieve uniform, symmetric compression across the fracture.

Scenario 2: Split-Depression Fractures

Split-depression fractures (Schatkzer II) are the most commonly presenting tibial plateau fracture pattern. Here, we prefer a formal open, anterolateral approach for direct assessment and visualization of the extent of the depression along with the joint articular surface.[29] Furthermore, we also recommend performing a formal open approach because of the high incidence of concomitant meniscal injury. Meniscal repair is an essential part of tibial plateau fracture repair and should not be ignored to perform percutaneous joint elevation and fixation. Buttress plating is the most common construct used to provide definitive stability.

Superficially, there are several options available for the initial skin incision and approach. The lazy S, the hockey stick, and a straight longitudinal incision centered over Gerdy tubercle have all been described.[29] Each has their advantages and disadvantages, and use should depend on surgeon familiarity.

Here, a 38-year-old man presented with a split-depression fracture after being struck by a motor vehicle while walking (**Fig. 3**A, B). CT revealed a more severe injury than led on by radiographs, with noted condylar widening, significant articular depression, and comminution (see **Fig. 3**C, D). Skin wrinkling was appreciated 5 days after the injury and the patient was taken to the operative room. An anterolateral approach was used. This approach differs from the classic hockey-stick approach because the proximal limb lies more proximal to the joint surface to allow for articular surface visualization. In addition, the distal limb is not as extensile to minimize deeper, soft tissue stripping. More importantly, on deeper dissection, the "L" portion of the approach is careful dissected and lifted from the capsule and bony surface as one, large subcutaneous flap, similar to that of the lateral approach to the calcaneus (see **Fig. 3**E). The senior author (KAE) prefers this approach because it not only allows for a more facile closure, but also has minimized soft tissue complications in his practice.[30,31]

The flap should be tagged with absorbable suture, which allows for easy retraction and visualization of deeper structures (see **Fig. 3**F).

Following submeniscal arthotomy, the meniscus should be identified and repaired and/or tagged in a vertical fashion, again to allow for retraction and visualization of the articular surface. These same sutures can be later used to stabilize the meniscus to any remaining tissue on the tibial side, or if none remains, can be passed and secured through the K-wire holes. At this juncture, with the fracture exposed, a laminar spreader can be used to book it open and assess the extent of joint depression (see **Fig. 3**G). After elevating the joint surface, provisional fixation can be placed to hold the split reduction in place. Although a recent biomechanical study has shown decreased rate of loss of reduction by placing drillable bone substitute before fixation, we still prefer to obtain and fluoroscopically confirm our articular reduction with provisional and definitive fixation before void filling.[32] Injectable calcium phosphate remains our void filling substitute of choice because it has been shown to have the highest compressive strength with minimal loss of reduction when compared with autograft, allograft, and calcium sulfate in clinical studies.[33–36]

After visually and fluoroscopically confirming the quality of the reduction, a periarticular, precontoured plate can be applied (see **Fig. 3**H). Plates larger than 3.5 mm are unnecessary because biomechanical studies have no shown no difference between the two sizes.[37] Furthermore, although it is certainly reasonable to place locking screws underneath the articular surface, if bone stock is adequate, distally, nonlocking fixation may be used. Repair of the meniscus, and appropriate opposition of the thick, subcutaneous flap should be carefully closed, with care paid to the corner of the incision. Following these steps, uneventful healing and good outcomes can be achieved (see **Fig. 3**I).

Scenario 3: Fracture-Dislocations

Fracture-dislocations of the tibial plateau indicate significant associated energy and warrant special attention. Even before planning definitive fixation, thorough and close monitoring of neurovascular status is required, and often soft tissue injury is more severe than indicated by the underlying bony pathology. Fracture-dislocations should warrant ABIs and frequent vascular examinations, especially with medial plateau fractures (Schatzker 4, Moore 1, **Fig. 4**A, B) and rim avulsion fractures (Moore 3, **Fig. 5**A, B), which are associated with at least a 10% incidence of associated neurovascular and/or ligamentous disruption.[38,39]

Schatzker IV and Moore 1 injuries essentially occur when the femoral condyle is driven down

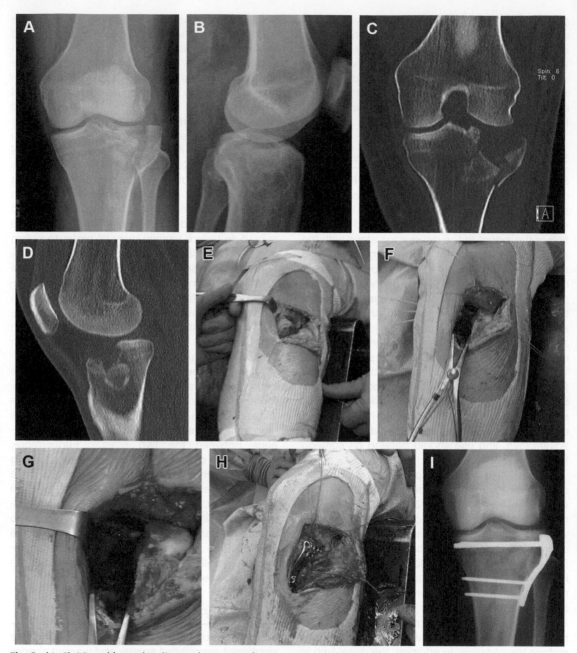

Fig. 3. (*A, B*) AP and lateral radiographs can mask a more severe degree of widening and depression that can be appreciated on CT (*C, D*). The senior author prefers a modified "L" incision and approach similar to the thick flap created for calcaneus fractures (*E*). Tagging the flap along with the meniscus allows for good visualization of the articular surface and fracture (*F*), which can be opened with a laminar spreader for proper assessment (*G*). Hardware placement before void filling is preferred to ensure and confirm anatomic reduction without the complication of excess substance (*H*). With appropriate meniscal repair, and closure, desired fracture healing and joint line restoration can be achieved (*I*).

into the tibia, effectively fracturing and shearing off the medial plateau. Here, a 44-year-old man fell off of a ladder, sustaining a fracture-dislocation (see **Fig. 4**A, B). Grossly unstable, with associated soft tissue swelling, there should be a low threshold to obtain temporary stabilization (see **Fig. 4**C, D).

Definitive fixation for this injury pattern can be applied in a step-wise process: interfragmentary screws between the condyles followed by buttress plating (see **Fig. 4**E, F). Surgical approach is dictated by plane of the fracture pattern. For medial plateau fractures in the coronal plane, a standard medial

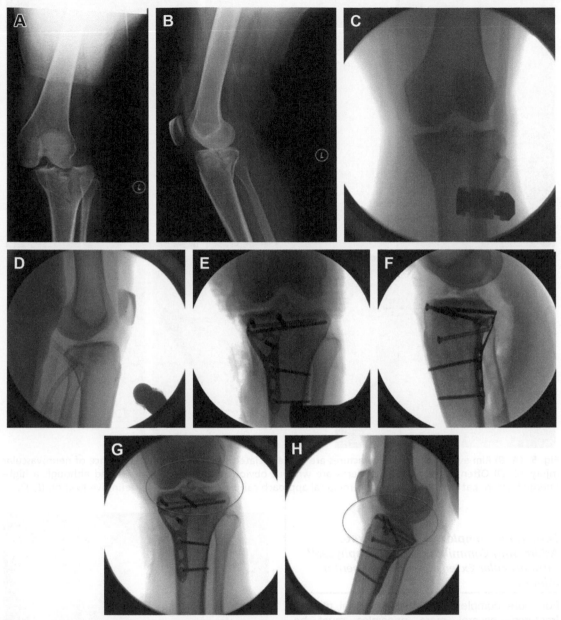

Fig. 4. Fracture-dislocations of the tibial plateau (*A, B*) are high-energy fractures commonly associated with neurovascular or ligamentous instability. There should be a low threshold to place an external fixator for gross instability (*C, D*). Fixation strategies should start with interfragmentary fixation between the condyles followed by buttress plating (*E, F*). Finally, before leaving the operating room, the affected limb should be stressed to assess for any ligamentous injury (*circles*), which is common (*G, H*).

approach can be used. However, for Moore 1 fractures where the fracture line is in the sagittal plane, creating a posteromedial fragment, the posteromedial approach working between the medial head of the gastrocnemius and the semimembranosus may offer an easier point of access for placing the buttress plate (see **Fig. 4**E, F).[40] Finally, an intraoperative ligamentous examination should be performed because it is not uncommon that ligamentous

reconstruction is required (and if so, it is typically fixed in a staged fashion) (see **Fig. 4**G, H).

Rim avulsion fractures (Moore 3) also carry a higher rate of associated neurovascular injury. This 67-year-old woman was a pedestrian struck who presented with concomitant peroneal nerve palsy (see **Fig. 5**A–D). A standard, anterolateral approach, as described previously, can be used to provide definitive fixation (see **Fig. 5**E, F).

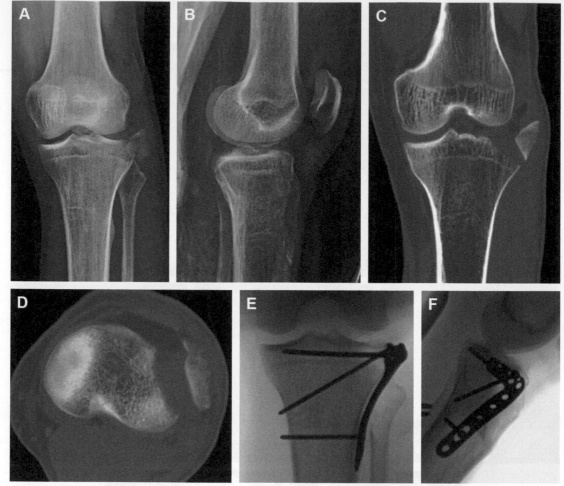

Fig. 5. (*A, B*) Rim avulsion (Moore 3) fractures are also associated with an increased incidence of neurovascular injury. (*C, D*) Often, these fracture patterns are without obvious joint line depression and although a high-energy fracture pattern, a standard, anterolateral approach can be used to provide definitive fixation (*E, F*).

Scenario 4: Complex, Bifocal Fractures, Addressing Comminution, Metadiaphyseal/Intra-articular Extension, and Segmental Injuries

For more complex, higher-energy tibial plateau fractures, several more principles must be considered.

- Be patient and wait for the soft tissues. Most of these fractures require temporary stabilization with an external fixator.
- Obtain CT after achieving length with external fixator.
- Leave the external fixator on, because it can serve as a valuable distractor to help maintain length (**Fig. 6**) and if an ex-fix is not on, have a femoral distractor ready and have a low threshold for use (**Fig. 7**).
- Do not hesitate to release compartments if compartment syndrome is suspected; have a low threshold for fasciotomies.

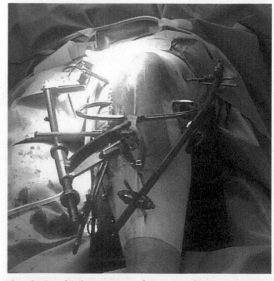

Fig. 6. For higher-energy fractures that are temporarily spanned, leaving the external fixator on during definitive fixation can offer an additional distraction tool that can be incredibly helpful.

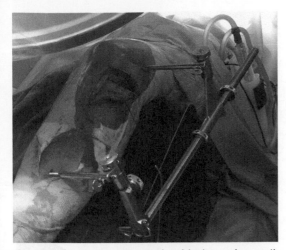

Fig. 7. A femoral distractor should always be available, and to obtain additional visualization, there should be a low threshold to place it.

- Multiple surgical approaches may be required.
- Do not be afraid to stage operations (ie, medial then lateral, or vice versa).
- For long, bifocal injuries that extend far distal or present as segmental injuries, additional fixation may be required to achieve desired level of stability.

In our first case example, a 22-year-old woman was ejected out of her motor vehicle. Her left lower extremity presented with obvious swelling and deformity with a tense calf. Initial radiographs revealed a comminuted tibial plateau fracture where the femur has driven itself into the proximal tibia (**Fig. 8**A, B). With increasing concern for compartment syndrome, the patient was taken to the operating room for compartment releases and stabilization with a spanning knee fixator, which achieved reduction, allowing for

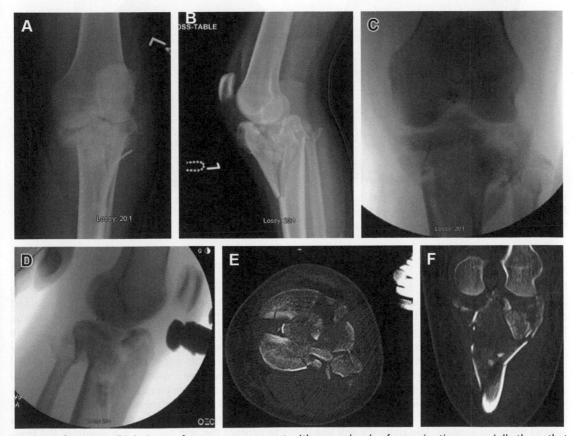

Fig. 8. High-energy tibial plateau fractures can present with severe levels of comminution, especially those that experience severe axial load of the femur into the proximal tibia (*A, B*). These fractures often require temporary stabilization with external fixation (*C, D*) and a CT should be obtained after ex-fix (*E–G*). With severe fracture patterns, staging each column is also acceptable, by starting with the easier side (*H, I*), allowing for the soft tissues to recover, and return to complete fixation (*J, K*).

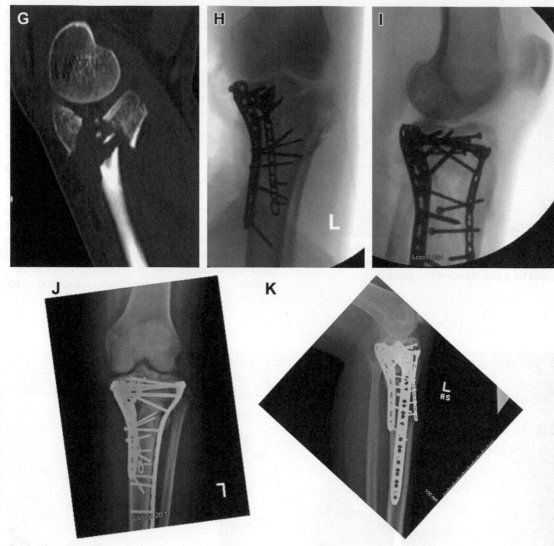

Fig. 8. (*continued*)

temporarily restored length (see **Fig. 8**C, D). Obtaining a CT after restoring length, one can better appreciate and understand the nature of the fracture (see **Fig. 8**E–G).

Analyzing the CT, the medial side appears to be in larger, more reconstructable fragments, and thus was fixed first (see **Fig. 8**H, I). Because of the severity of the injury and the time required to reconstruct only the medial side, the fasciotomies were closed and a negative pressure wound dressing applied. The patient's soft tissue status was closely monitored and when skin wrinkling was seen, the patient was brought to complete reconstruction of the lateral side (see **Fig. 8**J, K).

In our next case, distal extension with a long area of metadiaphyseal comminution presented a more difficult challenge. This type of bifocal injury often requires additional fixation to achieve appropriate stability. This 67-year-old woman after motor vehicle accident presented with a tibial plateau fracture with distal metadiaphyseal extension and significant comminution. Despite plate application via minimally invasive percutaneous plate osteosynthesis (MIPPO) technique to protect the soft tissues, the length of the fracture comminution still remained unstable (**Fig. 9**A–C). Dual plating provided a more stable construct for this long segment of comminuted bone (see **Fig. 9**D, E).

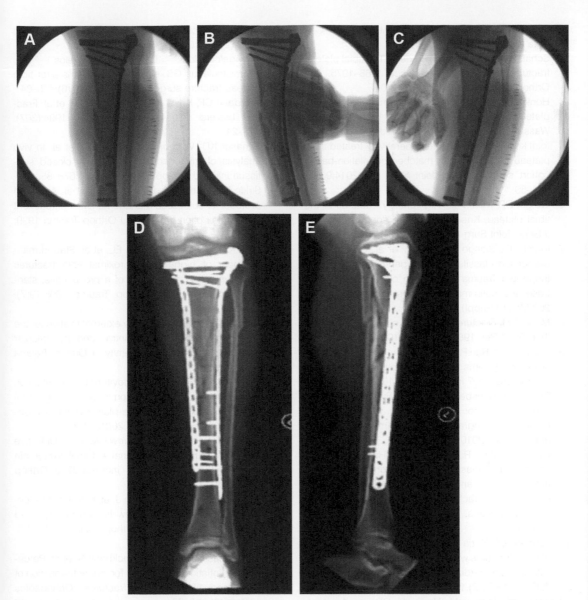

Fig. 9. Plateau fractures that present with long, distal extension of metadiaphyseal comminution offer a unique challenge. These bifocal injuries often remain unstable even following initial plate fixation (A–C), and at times require additional plating to achieve desired stability (D, E).

SUMMARY

Tibial plateau fracture presents in a wide range of fracture patterns, associated injuries, and soft tissue concerns. General principles along with a step-wise approach can be applied to every fracture and anatomic reduction and restoration of the mechanical axis. Definitive fixation should match the nature of each fracture pattern with the goals of always respecting the soft tissues. There should be a low threshold to apply a staged treatment protocol with a temporary external fixator in order for the soft tissues to optimize. CT scans offer detailed information about the fracture pattern, and in higher-energy fractures, should be obtained after restoring length and stability. Understanding the nature of the injury and applying the appropriate fixation to achieve ideal reduction and stability can be achieved, even in the most complex fracture patterns, with a desired clinical result.

REFERENCES

1. Allgoewer M, Mueller ME, Schenk R, et al. Biomechanical principles of the use of metal in bone. Langenbecks Arch Klin Chir Ver Dtsch Z Chir 1963;305: 1–14 [in German].

2. Mueller ME. Principles of osteosynthesis. Helv Chir Acta 1961;28:198–206 [in French].

3. Schatzker J, McBroom R, Bruce D. The tibial plateau fracture. The Toronto experience 1968–1975. Clin Orthop Relat Res 1979;(138):94–104.

4. Honkonen SE. Degenerative arthritis after tibial plateau fractures. J Orthop Trauma 1995;9(4):273–7.

5. Wasserstein D, Henry P, Paterson JM, et al. Risk of total knee arthroplasty after operatively treated tibial plateau fracture: a matched-population-based cohort study. J Bone Joint Surg Am 2014;96(2):144–50.

6. Weigel DP, Marsh JL. High-energy fractures of the tibial plateau. Knee function after longer follow-up. J Bone Joint Surg Am 2002;84-A(9):1541–51.

7. Marsh JL, Slongo TF, Agel J, et al. Fracture and dislocation classification compendium - 2007: Orthopaedic Trauma Association classification, database and outcomes committee. J Orthop Trauma 2007;21(10 Suppl):S1–133.

8. Moore TM. Fracture–dislocation of the knee. Clin Orthop Relat Res 1981;(156):128–40.

9. Maripuri SN, Rao P, Manoj-Thomas A, et al. The classification systems for tibial plateau fractures: how reliable are they? Injury 2008;39(10):1216–21.

10. Brunner A, Horisberger M, Ulmar B, et al. Classification systems for tibial plateau fractures; does computed tomography scanning improve their reliability? Injury 2010;41(2):173–8.

11. Patange Subba Rao SP, Lewis J, Haddad Z, et al. Three-column classification and Schatzker classification: a three- and two-dimensional computed tomography characterisation and analysis of tibial plateau fractures. Eur J Orthop Surg 2014;24(7):1263–70.

12. Forman JM, Karia RJ, Davidovitch RI, et al. Tibial plateau fractures with and without meniscus tear: results of a standardized treatment protocol. Bull Hosp Jt Dis 2013;71(2):144–51.

13. Spiro AS, Regier M, Novo de Oliveira A, et al. The degree of articular depression as a predictor of soft-tissue injuries in tibial plateau fracture. Knee Surg Sports Traumatol Arthrosc 2013;21(3):564–70.

14. Stannard JP, Lopez R, Volgas D. Soft tissue injury of the knee after tibial plateau fractures. J Knee Surg 2010;23(4):187–92.

15. Wagner HE, Jakob RP. Plate osteosynthesis in bicondylar fractures of the tibial head. Unfallchirurg 1986;89(7):304–11 [in German].

16. Barei DP, Nork SE, Mills WJ, et al. Complications associated with internal fixation of high-energy bicondylar tibial plateau fractures utilizing a two-incision technique. J Orthop Trauma 2004;18(10):649–57.

17. Lachiewicz PF, Funcik T. Factors influencing the results of open reduction and internal fixation of tibial plateau fractures. Clin Orthop Relat Res 1990;(259):210–5.

18. Papagelopoulos PJ, Partsinevelos AA, Themistocleous GS, et al. Complications after tibia plateau fracture surgery. Injury 2006;37(6):475–84.

19. Giordano CP, Koval KJ, Zuckerman JD, et al. Fracture blisters. Clin Orthop Relat Res 1994;(307):214–21.

20. Schaser KD, Vollmar B, Menger MD, et al. In vivo analysis of microcirculation following closed soft-tissue injury. J Orthop Res 1999;17(5):678–85.

21. Sirkin M, Sanders R, DiPasquale T, et al. A staged protocol for soft tissue management in the treatment of complex pilon fractures. J Orthop Trauma 1999;13(2):78–84.

22. Egol KA, Tejwani NC, Capla EL, et al. Staged management of high-energy proximal tibia fractures (OTA types 41): the results of a prospective, standardized protocol. J Orthop Trauma 2005;19(7):448–55 [discussion: 456].

23. Haidukewych GJ. Temporary external fixation for the management of complex intra- and periarticular fractures of the lower extremity. J Orthop Trauma 2002;16(9):678–85.

24. Laible C, Earl-Royal E, Davidovitch R, et al. Infection after spanning external fixation for high-energy tibial plateau fractures: is pin site-plate overlap a problem? J Orthop Trauma 2012;26(2):92–7.

25. Shah CM, Babb PE, McAndrew CM, et al. Definitive plates overlapping provisional external fixator pin sites: is the infection risk increased? J Orthop Trauma 2014;28(9):518–22.

26. Koval KJ, Sanders R, Borrelli J, et al. Indirect reduction and percutaneous screw fixation of displaced tibial plateau fractures. J Orthop Trauma 1992;6(3):340–6.

27. Hahnhaussen J, Hak DJ, Weckbach S, et al. Percutaneous inflation osteoplasty for indirect reduction of depressed tibial plateau fractures. Orthopedics 2012;35(9):768–72.

28. Vendeuvre T, Babusiaux D, Breque C, et al. Tuberoplasty: minimally invasive osteosynthesis technique for tibial plateau fractures. Orthop Traumatol Surg Res 2013;99(4 Suppl):S267–72.

29. Kandemir U, Maclean J. Surgical approaches for tibial plateau fractures. J Knee Surg 2014;27(1):21–9.

30. Egol KA, Su E, Tejwani NC, et al. Treatment of complex tibial plateau fractures using the less invasive stabilization system plate: clinical experience and a laboratory comparison with double plating. J Trauma 2004;57(2):340–6.

31. Urruela AM, Davidovitch R, Karia R, et al. Results following operative treatment of tibial plateau fractures. J Knee Surg 2013;26(3):161–5.

32. Hoelscher-Doht S, Jordan MC, Bonhoff C, et al. Bone substitute first or screws first? A biomechanical

comparison of two operative techniques for tibial-head depression fractures. J Orthop Sci 2014; 19(6):978–83.

33. Berkes MB, Little MT, Schottel PC, et al. Outcomes of Schatzker II tibial plateau fracture open reduction internal fixation using structural bone allograft. J Orthop Trauma 2014;28(2):97–102.

34. Goff T, Kanakaris NK, Giannoudis PV. Use of bone graft substitutes in the management of tibial plateau fractures. Injury 2013;44(Suppl 1):S86–94.

35. McDonald E, Chu T, Tufaga M, et al. Tibial plateau fracture repairs augmented with calcium phosphate cement have higher in situ fatigue strength than those with autograft. J Orthop Trauma 2011;25(2): 90–5.

36. Ozturkmen Y, Caniklioglu M, Karamehmetoglu M, et al. Calcium phosphate cement augmentation in the treatment of depressed tibial plateau fractures with open reduction and internal fixation. Acta Orthop Traumatol Turc 2010;44(4):262–9.

37. Hasan S, Ayalon OB, Yoon RS, et al. A biomechanical comparison between locked 3.5-mm plates and 4.5-mm plates for the treatment of simple bicondylar tibial plateau fractures: is bigger necessarily better? J Orthop Traumatol 2014;15(2):123–9.

38. Berkson EM, Virkus WW. High-energy tibial plateau fractures. J Am Acad Orthop Surg 2006;14(1):20–31.

39. Koval KJ, Helfet DL. Tibial plateau fractures: evaluation and treatment. J Am Acad Orthop Surg 1995; 3(2):86–94.

40. Fakler JK, Ryzewicz M, Hartshorn C, et al. Optimizing the management of Moore type I posteromedial split fracture dislocations of the tibial head: description of the Lobenhoffer approach. J Orthop Trauma 2007;21(5):330–6.

Upper Extremity

Preface

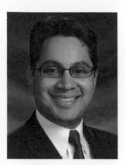

Asif M. Ilyas, MD
Editor

In this issue of the *Orthopedic Clinics of North America*, we present several interesting articles in the Upper Extremity section reviewing a broad range of topics.

There has been growing interest in the use of acellular human dermal allograft in various orthopedic applications. In particular, these grafts have been shown to help manage various challenging tendon deficiencies where they can be used to either augment or bridge soft tissue defects. Acevedo and colleagues provide a detailed review of the background and indications for this allograft in shoulder and elbow surgery.

The utilization of shoulder arthroplasty continues to grow in North America and this growth has resulted in the identification of a number of surgical challenges. One such challenge is the management of glenoid bone loss, which can compromise glenoid component fixation. Abboud and colleagues present a detailed review of the problem and of the literature and present their technique to manage this challenge.

Perioperative pain management is an essential aspect of orthopedic surgery. This is particularly true in hand surgery, where a number of modalities can be utilized to manage pain both perioperatively and postoperatively. In particular, how the surgical pain is managed perioperatively directly impacts how the surgery is performed. For instance, whether the surgery requires general anesthesia, regional anesthesia, sedation, or only local infiltration of anesthetics is predicated on the modality utilized. Ketonis and colleagues provide a detailed review of perioperative pain anesthetic modalities as well as the latest postoperative pain management strategies.

Asif M. Ilyas, MD
Hand & Upper Extremity Surgery
Rothman Institute
Thomas Jefferson University
925 Chestnut Street
Philadelphia, PA 19107, USA

E-mail address:
asif.ilyas@rothmaninstitute.com

Orthop Clin N Am 46 (2015) xvii
http://dx.doi.org/10.1016/j.ocl.2015.03.003
0030-5898/15/$ – see front matter © 2015 Published by Elsevier Inc.

Orthopedic Applications of Acellular Human Dermal Allograft for Shoulder and Elbow Surgery

CrossMark

Daniel C. Acevedo, MD*, Brett Shore, MD,
Raffy Mirzayan, MD

KEYWORDS

- Dermal allograft • Acellular dermal graft • Rotator cuff augmentation • Extracellular matrix
- Acromioclavicular joint injuries • Distal biceps ruptures • Tendon injuries of the shoulder and elbow
- Tendon augmentation

KEY POINTS

- Allograft augmentation for tissue repair should be biologic, sterile, non-inflammatory, and have good suture pullout strength.
- Human dermal allograft is an extracellular collagen matrix that acts as a collagen scaffold for host cell repopulation and integration.
- Surgical applications for human dermal allografts are evolving.

INTRODUCTION

Tendon injuries to the upper extremity can be challenging to treat. Injuries to the shoulder and elbow (ie, rotator cuff tears, distal biceps ruptures, pectoralis major ruptures) are due to abnormal or degenerative tendons. Surgical repair of tendon injuries in the upper extremity can be complicated by early failure due to inadequate repair (mostly attributed to inadequate suture-tendon interface strength) or late failure (mostly attributable to inadequate tendon to bone healing). Massive rotator cuff tears can have failure rates greater than 90%.[1] Failure of surgical repair of any tendon in the upper extremity can be related to many factors, namely tendon quality and the patient's own biology.

Augmentation of tendons with xenograft collagen matrices has been reported in the literature with poor outcomes. Ianotti[2] reported unfavorable outcomes with the use of a porcine submucosal patch in rotator cuff repairs. Walton and colleagues[3] reported severe inflammatory reactions to the porcine patch, which resulted in the total abandonment of grafts in rotator cuff repair augmentation. Ultimately, the ideal augmentation graft should be biologic, sterile, noninflammatory, and have excellent suture pullout strength.

The use of extracellular matrices for augmentation of soft tissue repairs in orthopedic surgery has gained recent interest in an attempt to improve healing and surgical outcomes. There are many commercially available dermal allografts and xenografts for use in orthopedic surgery. These soft tissue grafts include human dermis, porcine dermis, porcine intestinal submucosa, and synthetic materials. While, there is a paucity of

---

Disclosures: R. Mirzayan, Royalties – Wolters Kluwer, Thieme, Research Grants – Arthrex, JRF, BioD LLC, Stocks – Cayenne Medical, ITS-US Implants, Alignmed. Dr D.C. Acevedo and Dr B. Shore have nothing to disclose.
Department of Orthopedic Surgery, Kaiser Permanente, Baldwin Park, 13652 Cantara St, Panorama City, CA 91402, USA
* Corresponding author.
E-mail address: AcevedoMD@gmail.com

Orthop Clin N Am 46 (2015) 377–388
http://dx.doi.org/10.1016/j.ocl.2015.02.006

evidence available in the literature regarding the long-term outcomes with the use of these products, the small amount of literature currently available shows that the early results are promising.[4–11] Many of the applications for the use of these soft tissue collagen matrices, particularly human dermal allograft, also referred to as acellular dermal matrix (ADM), continue to evolve. Human dermal allograft is an extracellular collagen matrix that has been shown to have tissue integration properties, in vivo revascularization, cellular incorporation, and excellent biomechanical properties that make it an attractive option for soft tissue augmentation procedures in orthopedics.[4–11] Surgeons who wish to use these products in their practice should be versed with the available products on the market, their potential uses, preparation, safety, and surgical techniques. There are other collagen matrices currently available on the market, such as xenograft small intestinal submucosa (SIS) and synthetic collagen matrices that are beyond the scope of this article. This review focuses on the properties, uses, and surgical applications for the use of human dermal allografts in shoulder and elbow surgery.

THE BASICS OF DERMAL ALLOGRAFT

Human dermal allograft is a decellularized piece of human dermis that is processed and sterilized using various techniques to allow for human use. The dermal allograft is an extracellular collagen matrix, which is designed to be a collagen scaffold for tissue integration from the host. The allograft was intended for use as an "onlay" on top of a repair or as a bridge between tissues. The allograft also can be "incorporated into the repair" and can serve to strengthen the suture-tendon interface. For the allograft to be successful, it needs to have the ability to allow the host cells to migrate into it and incorporate themselves into the graft. The decellularization of human dermis is intended to remove the donor cells from the tissue, which may allow for the recipient cells to repopulate the graft faster and thus potentially allow for faster incorporation and revascularization, all while minimizing the risk of rejection and/or an inflammatory response. In theory, it provides a clean and cell-free scaffold. This decellularization process, however, may affect the biomechanical strength of the graft. Many available allografts have different levels of decellularization, although the ideal percentage of residual donor cells in the graft is unknown.

Dermal allografts, much like other extracellular collagen matrix scaffolds, elicit a histologic and a cytologic response to the tissues. Because it is an implantable product, the sterility of each product must be considered. Sterilization techniques for dermal allograft typically involve varying doses of radiation before packaging. Some available allografts are not sterilized. The clinical significance is currently unknown, but most implantable devices in orthopedics are sterilized before use. The biomechanical properties of each allograft may vary due to sterilization, preparation, storage, hydration, and methods of decellularization. These processes may affect the ability of the allograft to remodel and incorporate into the repair. The time frames of remodeling, incorporation, and degradation are currently not well understood for most dermal allograft products on the market at this time. Dermal allograft is an attractive option for tendon augmentation because it was shown to have superior suture pullout strength when used to augment rotator cuff repairs.[12]

Options for Acellular Dermal Matrices

When selecting the proper allograft to use in practice, some important factors regarding ADM should be considered (**Table 1**). Clinically applicable ADM products should be biocompatible, available in a range of sizes and thicknesses, have excellent suture retention properties, easy preparation, easy surgical handling, moderate costs, and ideally have some evidence-based support in the literature. Although clinical studies are currently lacking, there are some data to support the use of ADM in rotator cuff repairs.[5,7,11,13]

There are 4 major ADMs available on the market at this time: ArthroFlex (LifeNet Health, Virginia Beach, VA), Graft Jacket (Wright Medical Technology, Memphis, TN), AlloPatch HD (MTF, Edison, NJ), and Matrix HD (RTI Surgical, Alachua, FL).

ArthroFlex is a human dermal allograft that is considered a sterile product. A patented decellularization process called "Matracell" is used to remove more than 97% of the DNA from the graft. This specialized process has no adverse effect on the biomechanical properties. ArthroFlex is stored at room temperature, is hydrated in the packaging, and has a quick preparation time (**Fig. 1**). It is available off the shelf in multiple sizes and thicknesses.

GRAFTJACKET uses a proprietary decellularization process that renders the graft acellular. This product is processed with aseptic techniques and must be stored in a refrigerator. Because it is dehydrated, it requires a 15-minute rehydration and preparation time before implantation. This particular ADM product is available in multiple sizes and thicknesses off the shelf (**Fig. 2**).

AlloPatch HD is an ADM that has a quick preparation time and is also stored at room temperature.

Table 1
Properties of available dermal allografts

Product	Material	Processing	Sterilization	Donor DNA Removal	Storage	Storage Solution	Preparation Time	Strengths	Weaknesses
ArthroFlex (LifeNet Health)	Human dermis	Matracel	Low temp Low dose Irradiation	>97%	Room temperature	Saline	<1 min	Room temperature storage, sterile, fast preparation time	Relatively new product
Graft Jacket (Wright Medical)	Human dermis	Proprietary	None/Aseptic	N/A	Refrigerator	Dehydrated	>15 min	Numerous published studies	Refrigerator storage, >15 min preparation time, not sterile
AlloPatch HD (MTF)	Human dermis	Aseptic	None/Aseptic	N/A	Room temperature	70% Ethanol	<5 min	Room temperature storage, hydrated	Ethanol storage, not sterile, low suture pullout strength
Matrix HD (RTI biologics)	Human dermis	Tutoplast	Irradiation	N/A	Room temperature	Dehydrated	>10 min	Room temperature storage, 5-y shelf life	>10 min preparation time, Tutoplast processing, irradiated

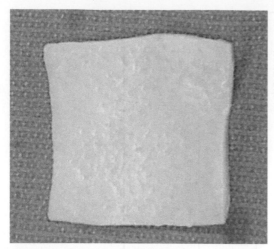

Fig. 1. ArthroFlex dermal allograft.

This product is processed with aseptic techniques and is stored in 70% ethanol.

Matrix HD is another ADM that is stored at room temperature and has a 5-year shelf life (**Fig. 3**). This product needs to be rehydrated and has an approximately 10-minute preparation time. This product undergoes a sterilization technique named "Tutoplast," which is a specialized chemical sterilization process that removes bacteria and pathogens from the graft without affecting the collagen structure. In addition, there is a low dose of gamma irradiation at the end of the process for final sterilization and packaging.

Safety of Human Dermal Allograft

The implantation of allograft tissues poses a risk of disease transmission, as well as rejection of the graft by the recipient. Initial use of extracellular matrix (ECM) products began with porcine SIS graft that was associated with poor results, including a 30% rate of severe inflammatory

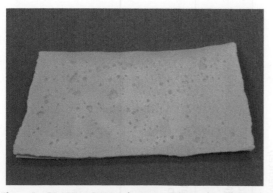

Fig. 2. GRAFTJACKET human dermal allograft. (Wright Medical Technology, Memphis, TN.)

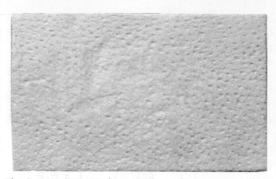

Fig. 3. Matrix™ HD dermal allograft. (*Courtesy of* RTI Surgical, Alachua, FL; with permission.)

response.[3] ADM products, however, have been shown to be safe in a several of clinical studies.[5,7,9–11,13]

The senior author (RM) has had personal experience with the use of ADM in more than 100 patients in the past 4 years. He has used ADM for augmentation of rotator cuff repair, distal biceps repairs, triceps repairs, pectoralis major repairs, elbow and knee capsule reconstructions, and acromioclavicular (AC) joint reconstruction, as well as patellar and quadriceps tendon ruptures. There have been no failures due to rejection, inflammatory reaction, or infection. Although this evidence is anecdotal, ADM appears to be safe for clinical use and long-term studies are currently in process at our institutions.

APPLICATIONS IN THE SHOULDER
Rotator Cuff Tears

Rotator cuff repairs in older patients can have a poor outcome due to failure of the tendon repair or inability to heal to bone. Retear rates have been shown in the literature to be higher than 90% for large and massive tear.[1] Multiple factors have been implicated as a role in rotator cuff repair failures, including smoking, age older than 63, massive tears, and fatty infiltration.[14] Suture pullout through the tendon is thought to be the most common method of failure.[7]

These problems sparked interest among surgeons to "augment" rotator cuff repairs. The use of extracellular collagen matrix for rotator cuff repairs is aimed at strengthening the repair by augmenting the suture-tendon interface, increasing the repair strength, and, thus, improving healing rates. Allografts have been shown to add to suture retention strength when used to augment a rotator cuff repair.[15] In addition, ADM grafts were stronger when compared with SIS grafts.[12] There have been multiple reports using ADM as a "bridging technique" in the repair of massive, retracted, irreparable rotator cuff tears by suturing the ADM graft to the rim of the retracted cuff tendon and repairing the ADM to the greater tuberosity. They demonstrated an arthroscopic technique with good clinical and radiographic (MRI) results.[8,13,16] Burkhead and colleagues[5] reported on a series of 17 patients with a massive or recurrent tear. ADM was used in an open rotator cuff repair as an "onlay." This study showed improved shoulder outcome scores and pain scores with no complications. Later studies introduced the use of ADM in an arthroscopic rotator cuff repair and showed good results with no adverse events related to the graft reported.[4,8,10,13,16]

There are currently 2 methods of using ADM for augmenting a rotator cuff repair: as an "onlay" on top of the repair to augment the repair and as a "bridge" to replace a deficient rotator cuff tendon. The indications for tendon augmentation with ADM as an "onlay" are advanced age, poor tendon quality, and for revision repairs. The rotator cuff surgery is performed arthroscopically. An anchor-based rotator cuff repair is performed using a standard posterior, posterolateral viewing, anterolateral working, and anterior portals. We prefer to use a SpeedBridge Repair (Arthrex, Naples, FL). The medial row anchors are placed first. One suture from each anchor is used to tie down the rotator cuff to the bone. The distance between the anchors is measured and the ADM is cut to a desired width and length. The fiber tape sutures are brought out through a cannula, placed through the ADM with a trochar/cutting needle, and the ADM is shuttled into the shoulder. A knotless lateral row anchor is then used to finish the cuff repair with the ADM on top of the tendon. The final construct is a double-row transosseous equivalent repair with an ADM "onlay." The ADM can increase the strength of the repair at the suture-tendon interface (**Fig. 4**).

Another technique uses the ADM as a "bridge" from the tendon to the bone, popularized by Bond and colleagues.[4] The indications for this procedure are massive retracted rotator cuff tears with low compliance for a standard repair and tendon-deficient rotator cuffs. In this procedure, the ADM is sutured to the most lateral edge of the rotator cuff either arthroscopically or through an open technique. The lateral edge of the ADM is repaired to the greater tuberosity. This technique serves as a "tendon replacement." The graft allows for cellular ingrowth of tendon from the medial rotator cuff to the bone. This technique has shown to be incorporated on postoperative MRI and histologic samples (**Fig. 5**).[13,16] This procedure can be performed open, although a more technically demanding arthroscopic technique also has been described by Snyder and colleagues.[8,16]

More recently, a new technique using small, preshaped pieces of ADM allograft to augment the repair of the rotator cuff by "incorporating" the ADM into the repair has been described by senior author, Raffy Mirzayan. Anchors are placed arthroscopically. The suture limbs from the anchors are retrieved with a suture grasper through a cannula one at a time to avoid tangling. The sutures are then passed through a small, preshaped ADM with a trochar/cutting needle, which is advanced into the shoulder with an arthroscopic knot pusher and placed under the cuff. The sutures are then passed through the rotator cuff tendon. The sutures are then individually brought back out the cannula and passed through another small preshaped ADM, which is advanced down the cannula and placed on top of the cuff. Essentially, the rotator cuff is "sandwiched" between 2 pieces of preshaped ADM. The preshaped ADM is easy to manage arthroscopically, and when incorporated into the repair, strengthens the suture-tendon

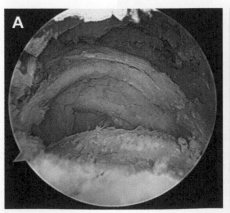
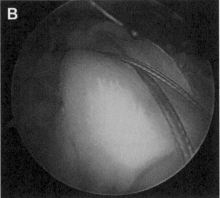

Fig. 4. (*A*) Arthroscopic view of a massive retracted rotator cuff tear. (*B*) Rotator cuff repair with dermal allograft as an "onlay" performed arthroscopically. (*Courtesy of* Namdari S, MD, Philadelphia, PA.)

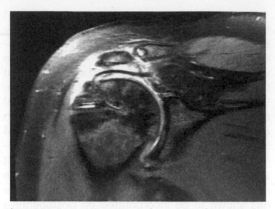

Fig. 5. Postoperative MRI arthrogram after a rotator cuff "bridging" procedure using dermal allograft. The ADM has healed to the rotator cuff medially and to the greater tuberosity.

interface (**Fig. 6**). This method serves 2 purposes: the ADM augments the suture-tendon interface and it assists with the healing of tendon to bone. Postoperative MRIs at 3 months in an ongoing series at our institution using preshaped ADM in 19 consecutive arthroscopic rotator cuff repairs have shown no (0%) retears at the repair site and 2 retears medial to the repair site (11%). This is a significantly lower retear rate than previously reported in the literature. The uses of ADM for rotator cuff repairs have promising potential; however, studies are needed to evaluate the long-term functional outcomes and healing rates.

SUPERIOR CAPSULAR RECONSTRUCTION FOR MASSIVE ROTATOR CUFF TEARS

Irreparable rotator cuff repairs can still pose a problem despite these augmentation techniques. Certain rotator cuff tears with retraction to the

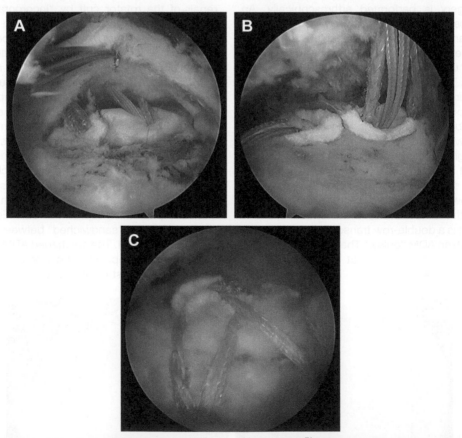

Fig. 6. (*A*) Two separate pieces of dermal allograft are used as BioWasher™ (LifeNet Health, Virginia Beach, VA). The FiberTape (Arthrex, Naples, FL) from each anchor is passed through each piece of allograft individually to lay directly on the greater tuberosity between the tendon and the bone. (*B*) After the fibertapes from each anchor are placed through the cuff, the fibertapes are passed through 2 additional allografts. The allograft lays on top of the tendon to complete the BioWasher™ Technique. The fiberwire strands from the anchor can also be passed through the grafts and tendon and used to tie knots medially, as in this example. (*C*) Final repair picture of a knotless double-row rotator cuff repair augmented with human dermal allograft BioWasher™.

glenoid margin, fatty atrophy, and advanced patient age cannot be mobilized enough for a repair or marginal convergence. A biomechanically proven concept, originally described by Mihata, has been introduced using ADM to reconstruct the superior capsule of the shoulder.[17] This procedure secures the ADM with anchors at the glenoid margin medially and at the greater tuberosity footprint laterally. This procedure restored the superior stability of the shoulder in a cadaveric study without altering the glenohumeral contact forces.[17] This "superior capsular reconstruction" can potentially restore the native kinematics of the shoulder, and prevent proximal migration of the humerus and subacromial impingement (**Fig. 7**).

This procedure can be performed both open and arthroscopically; however, visualization may be better arthroscopically. The size of the defect is measured and the appropriate-sized ADM, with a thickness greater than 2 mm is cut and prepared on the back table. FiberLink (Arthrex, Naples, FL) sutures are luggage tagged on the lateral edge of the graft to be repaired to the greater tuberosity on the back table. Three to 4 glenoid anchors are placed percutaneously into the superior glenoid. The sutures are then brought out of a lateral cannula systematically to prevent tangling. The sutures are passed through the ADM graft outside of the shoulder joint with a trochar/cutting needle. An arthroscopic knot pusher is used to advance the graft down the cannula and then reduce it to the glenoid. The sutures are tied to secure the graft to the glenoid. The sutures pre-placed in the graft for the lateral row are then secured to the greater tuberosity with additional anchors. There are currently no clinical studies evaluating the outcomes of this new procedure; however, it merits promise as a potential solution for a complex shoulder problem.

LATISSIMUS DORSI TENDON TRANSFERS

Tendon transfers for the upper extremity have been described for the treatment of massive and irreparable rotator cuff tears.[18] Latissimus dorsi tendon transfer serves as a viable surgical option for this complex problem with good long-term results.[19] This procedure can offer pain relief and improved functional outcomes with regard to forward elevation, external rotation, and strength. Functional results can be variable. Patient selection is important, as poor results have been demonstrated with deltoid dysfunction and in patients with subscapularis dysfunction.[18] This is a procedure that can be technically demanding due to the thin quality of the native latissimus dorsi tendon. Suturing the tendon with nonabsorbable sutures in a Krakow-type fashion is the standard suturing technique for the tendon. The tendon is

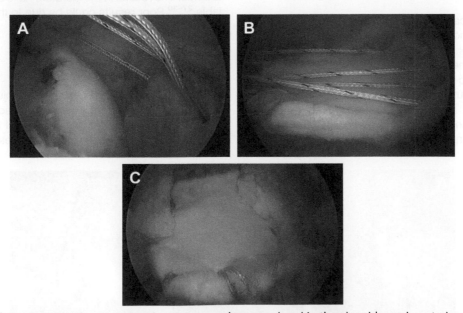

Fig. 7. (*A*) Superior capsular reconstruction. Suture anchors are placed in the glenoid margin anterior superiorly and posterior superiorly. (*B*) The ADM is shuttled into the shoulder through an arthroscopic cannula and secured to the glenoid with suture knots. (*C*) The lateral edge of the ADM is anchored to the greater tuberosity using fiberlink sutures and 2 knotless anchors. The anterior and posterior margins of the graft were sown to residual rotator cuff using free sutures passed with a suture passer to complete the superior capsule reconstruction.

then transferred under the deltoid to cover the greater tuberosity. Techniques can vary, but the latissimus is sutured anteriorly to the subscapularis, laterally into the greater tuberosity through transosseous sutures or anchors, and medially to the remnant of the rotator cuff if possible.

Failure of the tendon to heal to the tuberosity is the main cause of failure, which has led some investigators to perform an osteotomy technique in an attempt to improve healing.[20] ADM can be used to augment the tendon to improve suture pullout strength and to assist with the healing of the tendon to the bone. The ADM is wrapped around and incorporated with Krakow stitches onto the tendon. In addition, it can add to the repair strength to the subscapularis anteriorly (**Fig. 8**).

PECTORALIS MAJOR TENDON REPAIR

Pectoralis major tendon ruptures are often seen in heavyweight lifters and in work injuries.[21] Surgical repair is indicated in patients who do not want to accept the loss of strength or the cosmetic deformity. Surgical repair can be difficult, particularly in chronic cases. The tendon is usually short and thin, which makes achieving a good repair difficult. Achilles and fascia lata allografts have been used to reinforce the tendon to augment the repair.[22,23] Augmenting the pectoralis major with allograft tendon can be technically demanding and may not allow for improved healing.

ADM can be used to augment the pectoralis major tendon and has been shown to be a viable option for augmentation.[6] The ADM is wrapped around the tendon and muscle belly. This allows sutures to be passed through the tendon and muscle without strangulating or placing undue tension onto the muscle, thus increasing the "effective tendon length" of the pectoralis. The ADM is incorporated into the repair, strengthening the suture-

tendon interface, and augmenting the potential healing of the tendon onto the bone (**Fig. 9**). This technique is performed open, as any standard pectoralis major tendon repair would be. The final fixation to the humeral bone can be achieved via bone tunnels, suture anchors, or a unicortical suture button.

BIOLOGIC GLENOID RESURFACING

Shoulder arthritis in the young and/or active patient can be a difficult problem to treat. The gold standard for surgical management of cuff intact glenohumeral arthritis is a total shoulder arthroplasty. Patients younger than 40 years or high-demand shoulders can pose a risk for glenoid loosening and the need for early revision of the arthroplasty. Alternative procedures to a conventional total shoulder for the young and active patient include hemiarthroplasty, biologic glenoid resurfacing, or the "ream and run" procedures.

Biologic glenoid resurfacing has been described using fascia lata, meniscal allograft, and dermal allograft (**Fig. 10**).[24] High failure rates have been reported with the use of meniscal allografts and acellular dermal matrices.[25] There was a report of foreign body reactions when ADM was used in this procedure, one of the only reports in the literature regarding this type of reaction.[26] Currently it is unclear if biologic resurfacing of the glenoid remains a good option for the treatment of shoulder arthritis. The results in the literature have been variable.[27–30] Poor results could be due to the nature of the disease or to the choice of graft.

ACROMIOCLAVICULAR JOINT RECONSTRUCTION

AC joint injuries are common shoulder injuries that can result in significant pain and a decrease in function of the shoulder girdle. Surgical intervention is often required for grade 3 injuries that fail

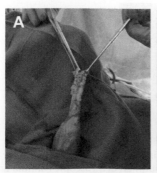
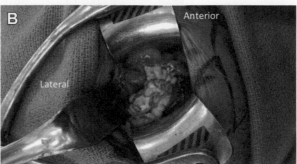

Fig. 8. (*A*) The ADM is sutured around the latissimus dorsi tendon. Krakow sutures are placed through the graft and tendon to incorporate the ADM. (*B*) The latissimus tendon is then transferred to the greater tuberosity and tied to the subscapularis tendon anteriorly.

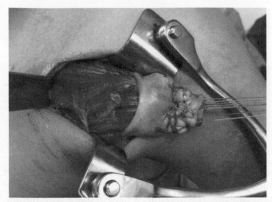

Fig. 9. A ruptured pectoralis major tendon wrapped with dermal allograft to strengthen the suture interface.

conservative treatment, and grade 4 to 6 injuries. Surgical intervention historically has been fraught with complications from the reconstructive techniques previously available.[31] Mazzocca and colleagues[32] recently described an anatomic reconstruction of the coracoclavicular ligaments with allograft tendon, which has become the most widely used surgical technique.

Current surgical techniques are aimed at reconstructing the coracoclavicular ligaments rather than the AC joint capsule. Biomechanical evidence has shown that the AC joint capsule plays a role in anterior-to-posterior stability in addition to vertical stability.[25,33–35] Adamson and colleagues[36] described a technique in which an intramedullary graft was used to reconstruct the AC joint capsule. This was shown in subsequent biomechanical studies to provide increased stability to the coracoclavicular joint reconstruction.[37,38] ADM, with its superior biomechanical properties and suture retention, can be used to reconstruct the AC ligaments as well as the capsule, thus improving anterior and posterior stability.

ADM as an intramedullary graft between the acromion and the clavicle has been used.[39] The graft is held in place with sutures passed through bone tunnels in the clavicle and the acromion, and tied over suture buttons. This is performed in addition to an anatomic coracoclavicular ligament reconstruction with allograft tendon with supplemental suture button fixation, and thus is referred to as an "AC/CC reconstruction." The ADM serves to stabilize the anterior-posterior stability, whereas the coracoclavicular ligament reconstruction stabilizes vertical stability. As opposed to allograft tendon, the ADM has favorable handling characteristics and allows sutures to be passed through it easily and quickly. It can be sized small enough, into a 1-cm square, which allows it to fit tightly as an interposition graft. The ADM has a high potential for cellular ingrowth and heals into a stable bridge across the AC joint. This technique has recently been described in the literature by the senior author (**Fig. 11**).[39] The senior author has performed this technique with ADM on 12 patients with good clinical and radiographic results. An outcome study is in process.

Elbow

The use of ADM in the elbow continues to evolve. There are not many described surgical techniques in the current literature. The use of ADM in the elbow may offer a solution to complex surgical problems in the future. We have used ADM for a few elbow procedures and discuss the use and the rationale in the following sections.

DISTAL BICEPS TENDON REPAIR

Distal biceps tendon ruptures usually occur from an eccentric muscle contraction with a load on the elbow. The distal biceps tendon is often bulbous and degenerative, requiring excision of

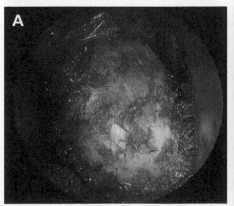
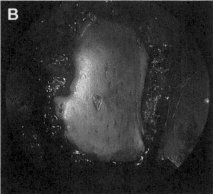

Fig. 10. (*A*) Glenoid of a young active patient with glenohumeral arthritis. (*B*) Biologic resurfacing of the glenoid with human dermal allograft. The graft is anchored with knotless suture anchors around the rim of the glenoid.

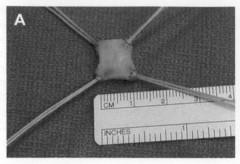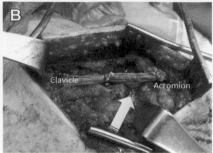

Fig. 11. (*A*) Dermal allograft is prepared with 4 nonabsorbable sutures at each corner. (*B*) Left shoulder AC joint reconstruction using the technique described by Lee and colleagues.[39] Dermal allograft (*yellow arrow*) used as an interpositional graft in the AC joint to reconstruct the AC joint capsule. The allograft is held in place with nonabsorbable sutures through the clavicle and acromion and tied over cortical buttons.

that portion of the tendon. Surgical repair is usually indicated to maintain supination and flexion strength in the extremity. Newer fixation techniques involving reduction of the tendon into a tunnel with fixation of a suture button and tenodesis screw have shown superior biomechanical pullout strength that have allowed an earlier functional recovery after surgical repair of distal biceps tendon ruptures.[40] The weak point in this repair is the tendon-bone tunnel junction. The biceps tendon is not only involved flexion of the elbow, which would be in line with the direction of pull with the tunnels, but it is also involved in forearm rotation. As the forearm is rotated, the tendon entrance

into the tunnel goes from 0° (full supination) to 90° (full pronation). This increases the amount of tension onto the tendon significantly as it enters the tunnel. By augmenting the tendon with ADM beyond the tunnel entrance, we can reduce the tension directed onto the tendon (**Fig. 12**). The senior author Raffy Mirzayan has used ADM to augment and strengthen degenerative distal biceps tendons in more than 40 single-incision distal biceps repairs using a cortical suture button and an interference screw ("tension slide" technique) with excellent results. There have been no retears. This method can allow for an even faster recovery with increased strength and potential

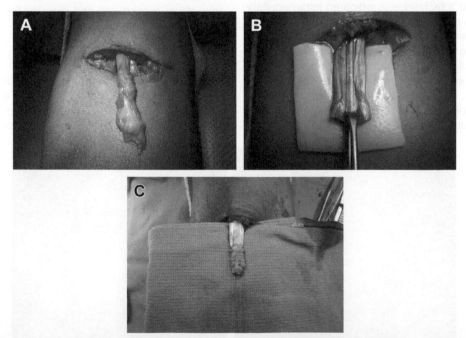

Fig. 12. (*A*) Distal biceps tendon rupture with degenerative distal tendon. (*B*) The ADM is wrapped around the distal edge of the graft. The graft is cut to size. (*C*) The ADM has been incorporated onto the distal biceps tendon with a locking suture.

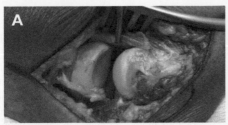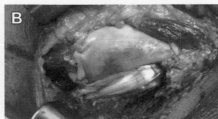

Fig. 13. (*A*) A patient with chronic PLRI. (*B*) LUCL reconstruction with capsular augmentation using dermal allograft.

for healing. During the rehabilitation period, the patients are allowed full active range of motion (AROM) for the first 4 weeks without a brace. Resistance exercises are started after 4 weeks and release to work as early as 2 to 3 months. The indications for use of ADM with distal biceps tendon ruptures are evolving. We believe this is best used with grossly degenerative and shredded tendons, chronic tears in which the tendon appears weakened, and in patients who wish to have an early return to work and function.

FUTURE APPLICATIONS IN ELBOW SURGERY

Elbow arthritis in the young and high-demand population can pose a challenge for surgical treatment. Interpositional arthroplasty is an option for this patient population.[41] Current graft options for "interposition" include Achilles tendon allograft and ADM. ADM has excellent handling properties and a superior suture retention strength, making it an attractive option for interpositional elbow arthroplasty. There is a lack of evidence supporting this procedure at this time. Another application in which the senior author Raffy Mirzayan has used ADM is for patients with posterolateral rotatory instability (PLRI). In addition to a deficient lateral ulnar collateral ligament (LUCL) the elbow capsule may be deficient or stretched from chronic posterior subluxation of the radial head. In patients with PLRI, the senior author performs a standard LUCL reconstruction with tendon allograft. If the capsule is deficient, an ADM is used to replace the deficient capsule by sewing the ADM to the tendon graft and the native elbow capsule (**Fig. 13**). This allows for increased stability to varus stress and prevents synovial fluid from leaking and bathing the tendon graft. Additional applications for ADM in the elbow are still evolving and outcome studies are currently lacking.

SUMMARY

ADM plays a role in a variety of applications for shoulder elbow surgery. There is a reasonable amount of evidence supporting its use along with

good short-term outcomes, particularly in the shoulder. ADM appears to be safe for implantation with a low risk of rejection, infection, or inflammatory response. Further research on the use of ADM is needed to determine long-term clinical outcomes.

REFERENCES

1. Galatz LM, Ball CM, Teefey SA, et al. The outcome and repair integrity of completely arthroscopically repaired large and massive rotator cuff tears. J Bone Joint Surg Am 2004;86:219–24.
2. Ianotti JP, Codsi MJ, Kwon YW, et al. Porcine small intestine submucosa augmentation of surgical repair of chronic two-tendon rotator cuff tears. A randomized, controlled trial. J Bone Joint Surg Am 2006; 88(6):1238–44.
3. Walton JR, Bowman NK, Khatib Y, et al. Restore orthobiologic implant: not recommended for augmentation of rotator cuff repairs. J Bone Joint Surg Am 2007;89(4):786–91.
4. Bond JL, Sopirak RM, Higgins J, et al. Arthroscopic replacement of massive, irreparable rotator cuff tears using GraftJacket allograft: technique and preliminary results. Arthroscopy 2008;24(4):403–9.
5. Burkhead WZ, Schiffern SC, Krishnan SG. Use of GraftJacket as an augmentation for massive rotator cuff tears. Semin Arthoplasty 2007;18(1):11–8.
6. Dehler T, Pennings AL, ElMaraghy AW. Dermal allograft reconstruction of a chronic pectoralis major tear. J Shoulder Elbow Surg 2013;22(10):e18–22.
7. Derwin KA, Badylak SF, Steinmann SP, et al. Extracellular matrix scaffold devices for rotator cuff repair. J Shoulder Elbow Surg 2010;19:467–76.
8. Dopirak R, Bond JL, Snyder SJ. Arthroscopic total rotator cuff replacement with an acellular dermal allograft matrix. Int J Shoulder Surg 2007;1(1):7–15.
9. Gupta AK, Hug K, Berkoff DJ, et al. Dermal tissue allograft for the repair of massive irreparable rotator cuff tears. Am J Sports Med 2012;40(1):141–7.
10. Modi A, Singh HP, Pandey R, et al. Management of irreparable rotator cuff tears with the GraftJacket allograft as an interpositional graft. Shoulder Elbow 2013;5:188–94.

11. Venouziou AI, Kokkalis ZT, Sotereanos DG. Human dermal allograft interposition for the reconstruction of massive irreparable rotator cuff tears. Am J Orthop 2013;42(2):63–70.

12. Barber FA, Herbert MA, Boothby MH. Ultimate tensile failure loads of a human dermal allograft rotator cuff augmentation. Arthroscopy 2008;24(1):20–4.

13. Wong I, Burns J, Snyder S. Arthroscopic GraftJacket repair of rotator cuff tears. J Shoulder Elbow Surg 2010;19(2 suppl):104–9.

14. Aleem AW, Brophy RH. Outcomes of rotator cuff surgery: what does the evidence tell us. Clin Sports Med 2012;31(4):665–74.

15. Beitzel K, Chowaniec DM, McCarthy MB, et al. Stability of double-row rotator cuff repair is not adversely affected by scaffold interposition between tendon and bone. Am J Sports Med 2012;40(5):1148–54.

16. Snyder SJ, Bond J. Technique for arthroscopic replacement of severely damaged rotator cuff using "Graft Jacket" allograft. Oper Tech Sports Med 2007;15:86–94.

17. Mihata T, McGarry MH, Pirolo JM, et al. Superior capsule reconstruction to restore superior stability in irreparable rotator cuff tears: a biomechanical cadaveric study. Am J Sports Med 2012;40(10):2248–55.

18. Omid R, Lee B. Tendon transfers for irreparable rotator cuff tears. J Am Acad Orthop Surg 2013;21:492–501.

19. Gerber C, Rahm SA, Catanzaro S, et al. Latissimus dorsi tendon transfer for treatment of irreparable posterosuperior rotator cuff tears: long term results at a minimum follow-up of ten years. J Bone Joint Surg Am 2013;95(21):1920–6.

20. Moursy M, Forstner R, Koller H, et al. Latissimus dorsi tendon transfer for irreparable rotator cuff tears: A modified technique to improve tendon transfer integrity. J Bone Joint Surg Am 2009; 2009(91):1924–31.

21. ElMaraghy AW, Devereaux MW. A systematic review and comprehensive classification of pectoralis major tears. J Shoulder Elbow Surg 2012;21:412–22.

22. Sikka RS, Neault M, Guanche CA. Reconstruction of the pectoralis major tendon with fascia lata allograft. Orthopedics 2005;28(10):1199–201.

23. Zachilli MA, Fowler JT, Owens BD. Allograft reconstruction of chronic pectoralis major tendon ruptures. J Surg Orthop Adv 2013;22(1):95–102.

24. Burkhead WZ, Krishnan SJ, Lin KC. Biologic resurfacing of the arthritic glenohumeral joint: historical review and current applications. J Shoulder Elbow Surg 2007;16(5 Suppl):S248–53.

25. Nicholson GP, Goldstein JL, Romeo AA, et al. Lateral meniscal allograft biologic glenoid arthroplasty in total shoulder arthroplasty for young shoulders with degenerative joint disease. J Shoul Elbow Surg 2007;16(5 suppl):S261–6.

26. Namdari S, Melnic C, Huffman GR. Foreign body reaction to acellular dermal matrix allograft in biologic glenoid resurfacing. Clin Orthop Relat Res 2013; 471(8):2455–8.

27. Strauss EJ, Verma NN, Salata MJ, et al. The high failure rate of biologic resurfacing of the glenoid in young patients with glenohumeral arthritis. J Shoulder Elbow Surg 2014;23(3):409–19.

28. Muh SJ, Sreit JJ, Shishani Y, et al. Biologic resurfacing of the glenoid with humeral head resurfacing for glenohumeral arthritis in the young patient. J Shoulder Elbow Surg 2014;23(8):e185–90.

29. Lee BK, Vaishnav S, Hatch R, et al. Biologic resurfacing of the glenoid with meniscal allograft: long-term results with minimum 2-year follow up. J Shoulder Elbow Surg 2013;22(2):253–60.

30. Hammond LC, Lin EC, Harwood DP, et al. Clinical outcomes of hemiarthroplasty and biological resurfacing in patients aged younger than 50 years. J Shoulder Elbow Surg 2013;22(10):1345–51.

31. Modi CS, Beazley J, Zywiel MG, et al. Controversies relating to the management of acromioclavicular joint dislocations. Bone Joint J 2013;95-B(12):1595–602.

32. Mazzocca A, Santangelo S, Johnson ST, et al. A biomechanical evaluation of an anatomical coracoclavicular ligament reconstruction. Am J Sports Med 2006;34:236–46.

33. Fukuda K, Craig EV, An KN, et al. Biomechanical study of the ligamentous system of the acromioclavicular joint. J Bone Joint Surg Am 1986;68:434–40.

34. Kliemkiwicz JJ, Williams GR, Sher JS, et al. The acromioclavicular capsule as a restraint to posterior translation of clavicle: a biomechanical analysis. J Shoulder Elbow Surg 1999;8:119–24.

35. Lee KW, Debski RE, Chen C. Functional evaluation of the ligaments at the acromioclavicular joint during anteroposterior and superoinferior translation. Am J Sports Med 1997;25:858–62.

36. Adamson GJ, Freedman JA, Lee TQ. Free tissue graft reconstruction of the acromioclavicular joint: a new technique. Tech Shoulder Elbow Surg 2008;9:193–8.

37. Freedman JA, Adamson GJ, Bui C, et al. Biomechanical evaluation of the acromioclavicular capsular ligaments and reconstruction with an intramedullary. Am J Sports Med 2010;38:958–64.

38. Gonzalez-Lomas G, Javidan P, Lin T, et al. Intramedullary acromioclavicular ligament reconstruction strengthens isolated coracoclavicular ligament reconstructions in acromioclavicular dislocations. Am J Sports Med 2010;38:2113–22.

39. Lee B, Acevedo D, Mirzayan R. Reconstruction of the acromioclavicular joint, its superior capsule, and coracoclavicular ligaments using an interpositional acellular dermal matrix and tibialis tendon allograft. Tech Shoulder Elbow Surg 2014;15(3):79–86.

40. Sethi PM, Tibone J. Distal biceps repair using cortical button fixation. Sports Med Arthrosc 2008;16(3):130–5.

41. Chen DD, Forsh DA, Hausman MR. Elbow interposition arthroplasty. Hand Clin 2011;27(2):187–97.

Glenoid Bone Loss in Anatomic Shoulder Arthroplasty
Literature Review and Surgical Technique

CrossMark

Daisuke Mori, MD[a], Joseph A. Abboud, MD[b,*],
Surena Namdari, MD, MSc[b], Gerald R. Williams, MD[b]

KEYWORDS

- C2 glenoid • Steptech • Augmented • All-polyethylene glenoid component
- Severe posterior glenoid bone loss

KEY POINTS

- Despite major advances in total shoulder arthroplasty, management of severe posterior glenoid bone loss remains controversial.
- Several companies have provided alternative treatment options for type C glenoids associated with posterior subluxation of the humeral head.
- Preoperative planning, proper selection of glenoid size, and recognition of the operative pitfalls are crucial for successful outcomes.

INTRODUCTION

With improvements in component design, technology, and surgical technique, total shoulder arthroplasty (TSA) is a highly successful surgical procedure for glenohumeral arthritis. However, lucent lines around the glenoid component and glenoid component loosening remain a major concern. Preoperative recognition of glenoid morphology and proper surgical planning are key factors for successful outcomes after surgical treatment of glenohumeral arthritis.[1–3]

The glenoid classification by Walch and colleagues[4] has been widely accepted for preoperative planning. Walch and colleagues classified glenoid morphology in primary glenohumeral arthritis into 5 types: In type A1, the humeral head is centered and minor glenoid erosion occurs

centrally. In type A2, the head is centered and major glenoid erosion occurs centrally. In type B1, the humeral head is subluxated posteriorly without glenoid erosion. In type B2, the humeral head is subluxated posteriorly and the glenoid has posterior erosion with the development of biconcavity. In type C, there is glenoid dysplasia or hypoplasia (retroversion >25°) with or without posterior wear. Among these types, the operative treatment of type B2 and C remains most controversial.[1–3]

The purpose of this article is to address the present operative strategies for B2 and C glenoids and to highlight the surgical technique and its pitfalls.

SURGICAL TREATMENT OF B2 GLENOID

Several treatment strategies have been reported for type B2 glenoids, such as asymmetric reaming,

Disclosures: Dr. Mori has no conflicts to disclose. Dr. Abboud is a consultant and designer for Integra Life Sciences. Dr. Namdari is consultant and receives royalties for product design from Miami Device Solutions and Bulletproof Bone Designs. Dr. Williams is consultant for Depuy, Mitek, and Tornier. He receives royalties for product design from Depuy, IMDS/Cleveland Clinic, and Lippincott.
[a] Department of Orthopaedic Surgery, Kyoto Shimogamo Hospital, 17 Shimogamo Higashimorigamecho, Skyo-ku, Kyoto 606-0866, Japan; [b] Rothman Institute at Thomas Jefferson University, 925 Chestnut Street, Philadelphia, PA 19107, USA
* Corresponding author.
E-mail address: abboudj@gmail.com

Orthop Clin N Am 46 (2015) 389–397
http://dx.doi.org/10.1016/j.ocl.2015.02.007

bone grafting, augmented components, and reversed TSA.

Asymmetric Reaming and Glenoid Resurfacing

With asymmetric reaming, it can be difficult to re-create normal glenoid version in cases of severe glenoid retroversion without removing substantial anterior bone. Sabesan and colleagues[5] demonstrated that correction of moderate to severe glenoid retroversion by asymmetric reaming cannot always be done with the use of a standard component, and if it is done, it will result in greater medialization of the joint line. In addition, Clavert and colleagues[6] have demonstrated that correction of greater than 15° of retroversion is not possible without violating the anterior subchondral bone or the glenoid vault with the anchoring points. Gillespie and colleagues[7] also have demonstrated that a 15° deformity has only a 50% chance of successful correction by anterior, eccentric reaming in a cadaveric model.

Basic study and clinical results of asymmetric reaming and glenoid implantation have been mixed. Most recently, Walch and colleagues[8] have demonstrated that violation of subchondral bone can lead to early glenoid radiolucency and failure. Study of the use of a standard glenoid component in the setting of a biconcave glenoid demonstrated high rates of complications.[9] Gillespie and colleagues[7] demonstrated that correction of as little as 10° of posterior glenoid wear by preferential anterior glenoid reaming results in significant narrowing of the glenoid anteroposterior distance by their cadaveric study. They also demonstrated that corrective glenoid reaming for wear of greater than 10° results in peg penetration in most glenoids and downsizing of glenoid size for most glenoids. On the other hand, Gerber and colleagues[10] showed that asymmetric reaming resulted in correction of posterior humeral subluxation in 21 of 23 patients (91%). Similarly, Habermeyer and colleagues[11] showed that, with asymmetric reaming and soft tissue balancing, the humeral head was maintained in a recentered position following surgical correction of glenoid morphology.

Ream and Run

"Ream and Run" is a specific procedure in which a humeral arthroplasty is performed for active patients in conjunction with concentric reaming of the glenoid bone to spherical concavity with a diameter of curvature 2 mm greater than that of the prosthetic humeral head. Clinton and colleagues[12] demonstrated that the ream and run can offer similar functional recovery to patients with TSA, although the time to recovery may be longer. Matsen and colleagues[13] presented that the ream and run substantially corrected the glenoid type in conjunction with B2 glenoid on the axial view radiographs. Gilmer and colleagues[14] concluded that the procedure appears to be best suited for older male patients with reasonable preoperative shoulder function without prior shoulder surgery, as an analysis of 176 consecutive cases after the procedure based on patient self-assessment, like the simple shoulder test. They also concluded that the type of glenoid had no significant effect on the outcome, and their patients had no problems with posterior glenohumeral instability, although a substantial number of the glenoids were posteriorly eroded and the humeral head was displaced into the posterior aspect of a biconcavity.

Bone Grafting

Studies of clinical and radiographic results of primary total shoulder replacement with an all-polyethylene glenoid component and autologous humeral head graft augmentation have demonstrated mixed results. Neer and Morrison[15] reported excellent results in 16 patients and satisfactory results in 3 patients, and no revision surgeries. No glenoid loosening or migration had occurred at a minimum follow-up of 2 years (average, 4.4 years). Steinmann and Cofield[16] reported that at a mean of 5 years postoperatively, 23 of 28 (82%) patients had satisfactory results after concomitant bone grafting and TSA. However, 15 patients (54%) demonstrated some degree of radiographic lucency, and 3 glenoids were radiographically loose at an average follow-up of 5.3 years. Hill and Norris[17] reviewed 17 TSAs at a mean of 70 months postoperatively that had undergone concomitant bone grafting to address glenoid erosion. Five (29%) of the grafts failed, resulting in requiring revision as a result of instability (2 patients). Sabesan and colleagues[18] reported that 10 of the 12 patients had graft incorporation without any resorption and 2 patients had minor bone graft resorption. Broken screws occurred in 2 of these 10 cases. Two patients, both of whom required revision surgery, had failure of fixation and of graft incorporation. These studies indicate that posterior subluxation can be corrected with glenoid bone grafting, but that the technique may be difficult to perform, generates inconsistent results, and may result in hardware complications and late graft failure in some cases.

Augmented Polyethylene Glenoid

When posterior bone loss is between 3 and 9 mm on the axial view, an augmented component can be used. It has been shown in a 3-dimensional surgical simulation that the use of an augmented component can allow complete correction of retroversion and minimize the effect of medialization.[5] Similarly, compared with a stepped, augmented component, retroversion greater or equal to 20° has been shown to make it difficult to place a pegged glenoid component perpendicular to the plane of the scapula by asymmetric reaming without center peg perforation.[19] In the senior author's practice (G.R.W.), a posteriorly augmented glenoid component is typically preferred in the setting of a B2 glenoid with between 3 mm and 9 mm of posterior bone loss.

Reverse Arthroplasty

At early follow-up, Mizuno and colleagues[20] reported successful clinical and radiographic results of reverse TSA for the treatment of primary osteoarthritis in patients with a biconcave glenoid without rotator cuff insufficiency. Despite this, reverse arthroplasty carries its own particular risks of complications and shortcomings. More data will be required to determine the indications of reverse arthroplasty in patients with posterior subluxation and posterior glenoid bone loss and an intact rotator cuff.

SURGICAL TREATMENT OF TYPE C GLENOIDS

Walch and colleagues[4] defined type C glenoid morphology as glenoid retroversion of greater than 25°. This type is most commonly associated with congenital or dysplastic development. Glenohumeral arthritis secondary to glenoid dysplasia appears to be relatively uncommon. Although type C glenoid is thought to be rare, some reports indicate that it may be more common than previously speculated and shoulder arthroplasty has proven to be a viable option. However, the choice of treatment options still remains controversial.[1,3,21–24] Bonnevialle and colleagues[21] reported marked improvement in pain scores, function, and outcome measures at a minimum 2-year follow-up in 9 patients treated with hemiarthroplasty for dysplasia. The authors concluded that hemiarthroplasty is a reliable management option for this patient population. On the other hand, Sperling and colleagues[23] reported that 3 of 4 patients treated with hemiarthroplasty underwent revision to TSA as a result of glenoid arthrosis at 16 months, 20 months, and 34 months. They concluded that hemiarthroplasty alone appears to be an unsatisfactory option for the treatment of dysplastic glenoid. Edwards and colleagues[22] demonstrated significant improvement in outcome measures at a mean of 37 months in 15 patients with primary osteoarthritis and type C glenoid treated with hemiarthroplasty or total arthroplasty. These successful results might be due to their criteria that glenoid resurfacing was 15 mm or greater of glenoid bone depth on axial computed tomography (CT).[23] However, in cases of severe dysplasia, the amount of bone available for fixation may be inadequate for standard fixation options. In these patients, the use of an inset bone-sparing glenoid component with a single, short peg may be helpful to avoid cortical penetration.[24]

Among shoulders with type C glenoids, there are certain shoulders whose humeral head does not remain centered on the surface of the glenoid and is posteriorly subluxated with regard to the surface of the glenoid, resulting in biconcavity; this may be defined as C2 glenoids (Michael Wiater, MD, personal communication, 2011) (**Fig. 1**). The posterior rotator cuff in a C2 glenoid is likely relatively short by virtue of the shorter distance between the origin and insertion of the muscles since birth. Hence, patients with C glenoids may lose internal rotation motion if correction of retroversion to neutral version is performed. Therefore, the author aims for correction of preoperative subluxation to the point where the humeral head is recentered on the surface of the native glenoid without necessarily completely correcting the version to neutral. Therefore, in the senior author's (G.R.W.) practice, a C2 glenoid (ie, biconcave) with 9 mm or greater of posterior bone loss is also an indication for a posteriorly augmented, stepped component, with the idea of correcting the biconcavity without complete correction of retroversion. Type C glenoids without posterior subluxation (C1) are less often corrected with an augmented component.

Surgical Indications

In the case of shoulders with 3 mm or greater of posterior wear, asymmetric reaming of the anterior glenoid (high side) is performed and a standard, pegged glenoid component is used. In shoulders with 5 mm of posterior wear, anterior reaming of 2 mm is undertaken and a 3-mm stepped component is used. In shoulders with 7 mm of posterior wear, anterior reaming of 2 mm is undertaken and a 5-mm stepped component is used. In shoulders with 9 mm of posterior wear, anterior reaming of 2 mm is undertaken and a 5-mm stepped component is used. In the cases of shoulders with greater than 9 mm of posterior wear, bone grafting is often indicated and a stepped component may not be appropriate. In rare cases of shoulders with inadequate peripheral or central bone to allow for placement of a pegged glenoid

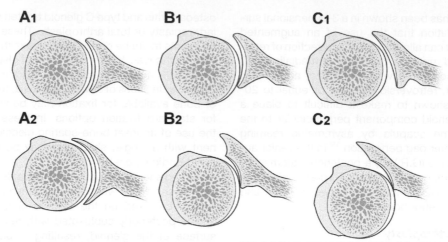

Fig. 1. A new classification of glenoid morphology. A1, type A1, centered humeral head with minor glenoid erosion. A2, type A2, centered humeral head with major glenoid erosion. B1, type B1, posterior subluxation with no erosion. B2, type B2, posterior subluxation with a biconcave glenoid. C1, type C1, severe retroversion and no posterior subluxation of humeral head. C2, type C2, severe retroversion with a biconcave glenoid and posterior subluxation of humeral head. (*Adapted from* Walch G, Badet R, Boulahia A, et al. Morphologic study of the glenoid in primary glenohumeral osteoarthritis. J Arthroplasty 1999;14(6):756–60; with permission.)

component (type C1 glenoids or revisions) or those thought to be at high risk for bone graft resorption and failure, a Mini Glenoid (Arthrosurface, Franklin, MA, USA) may be used.

These recommendations are only guidelines based on experience. In addition, it is important to note that the glenoid deficiency is 3-dimensional and includes differences in inferior tilt as well as anterior and posterior role. The 3-dimensional aspect of the deformity is difficult to appreciate without 3-dimensional CT imaging and application of software that can assist the surgeon in the appropriate placement of the component in all 3 planes. Multiple software programs currently exist to help achieve anatomic correction, but an in-depth discussion of this topic is beyond the scope of this article.

Surgical Technique

A standard deltopectoral approach is used. The superficial and deep dissections have been described in detail previously.[25] Current preference for subscapularis management is a lesser tuberosity osteotomy.

Preoperative Planning, Sizer Pin Guide Placement, and Sizing

Planned step height is determined based on the preoperative CT scan. If a preoperative preparation software system is available to the surgeon, it is helpful—particularly in cases of severe deformity. Iannotti and colleagues[19,27] demonstrated

that use of a preoperative planning tool based on CT scans provides more accurate placement of the component. Experience with these types of planning tools is currently not extensive but is increasing. In the future, this type of preoperative and intraoperative assistance in the placement of glenoid components in cases of glenoid bone loss is likely to be common.

In the absence of a preoperative planning tool, it is important for the surgeon to use the 3-dimensional CT scan to appreciate the glenoid deformity in all 3 planes. The most obvious plane is the axial plane. However, the coronal and sagittal planes are also important. Typically, posteriorly biconcave glenoids also demonstrate variable superior tilt in the coronal plane and posterior tilt in the sagittal plane. If, for example, the preoperative CT shows 5 mm of posterior bone loss on the axial cuts, a sizer pin guide with a 5-mm posterior buildup is selected so that, with 2 mm of anterior reaming, a 3-mm posterior step can be created for insertion of a 3-mm posteriorly augmented component (**Fig. 2**). The surgeon should also be cognizant of any superior or posterior tilt seen on the preoperative CT scan and adjust the direction of the pin accordingly.

When the surgeon is satisfied with the entry point and angle of insertion of the guide pin, the 2.5-mm breakaway guide pin is drilled into position through the curved handle/sizer pin guide assembly (**Fig. 3**A). This guide directs the guide pin in a manner to allow for preferential reaming of 2 mm of bone anteriorly. When the guide pin is driven

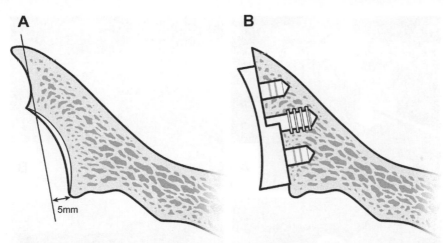

Fig. 2. (*A*) A black line is drawn on the anterior native glenoid. The amount of bone loss is measured by the distance between the line and posterior glenoid edge on the axial CT view. This case shows 5 mm of posterior glenoid bone loss. (*B*) A 3-mm StepTech component is inserted on the glenoid.

across the glenoid fossa, the distance between the glenoid face and the far cortex is ensured to be sufficient to allow for placement of the glenoid component without perforation of the central peg. Before drilling over this wire, the surgeon can often feel the tip of the guide pin anteriorly with digital palpation and confirm that the direction of the pin is appropriate. Most recently, the author made use of image analysis software (Ortho Vis; Cleveland Clinic, OH, USA) and Glenoid Smart Bone-Pin Trajectory instruments (custom shoulder solution) to allow for improved preoperative planning and proper intraoperative glenoid component preparation and placement.

Anterior Reaming

The anterior half of the glenoid is reamed until the reamed surface is even with the guide pin in the center of the glenoid surface (see **Fig. 3**B), typically resulting in approximately 2 mm of anterior glenoid reaming. In the system that is currently used, the anterior glenoid can be reamed in 2 stages—centrally and peripherally—or in one stage. Two-stage reaming is particularly useful in larger glenoids (ie, greater than size 48) because the one-stage reamer can be large and difficult to maneuver onto the glenoid surface over the guide pin (see **Fig. 3**C). The surgeon should ream the anterior glenoid side until the anterior half of the glenoid, up to the mid portion of the glenoid, has a concentric surface. Care should be taken to ensure that the anterior reamed surface is devoid of any prominent edges or any adherent soft tissue that might prevent complete seating of the posterior preparation guide or final component.

Posterior Preparation

Once the anterior glenoid surface has been prepared, the guide pin is drilled over with the central drill and the guide pin is removed. The posterior preparation guide for the appropriate step size is inserted into the central drill hole, impacted into position, and fixed with 2 stabilizing pins (see **Fig. 3**D). The posterior glenoid is then prepared with a combination of a burr and a vibratory rasp, using the anteriorly placed guide as a template. First, the sclerotic bone of the posterior glenoid is removed to a rough depth of 2 mm using a burr (see **Fig. 3**E). The vibratory rasp with the selected step size is then used to precisely create the posterior step. The rasp is seated on the anterior surface of the rasp guide to maintain the targeted depth of reaming (see **Fig. 3**F). Small and large rasps are available in each step size. The larger one is most useful in glenoid sizes of 48 mm and larger. The smaller rasp is intended for the smaller sized glenoids but may also be useful in the larger glenoids at the most superior and inferior portions of the glenoid where the anteroposterior dimensions of the glenoid are smaller. The rasp will create a step that is sloped from the posterior periphery of the glenoid toward the center. During inferior instrumentation with the rasp or burr, a blunt Hohmann retractor is placed on the inferior scapular neck to protect the axillary nerve.

After posterior reaming is completed, an estimate of the depth of the step is made using a free guide pin. The tip of the pin is placed on the reamed posterior surface and a clamp is placed on the pin, where it meets the inferior

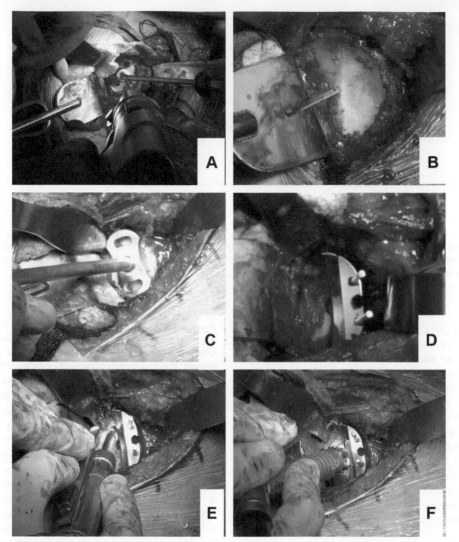

Fig. 3. Right shoulder. (*A*) A sizer pin guide with posterior buildup is set on the glenoid surface and a 2.5-mm breakaway guide pin is inserted through the curved handle/sizer pin guide assembly. (*B*) A right shoulder. The anterior half of the glenoid is reamed about 2 mm. (*C*) A low-profile peripheral reamer is manually rotated to clean up the edge of anterior reamed surface. (*D*) A rasp guide is seated on the anterior portion of the reamed glenoid with 2 pins. (*E*) Initially, the surgeon should remove the posterior half of the glenoid with a bur. (*F*) The matching size vibratory rasp is on an anterior rasp guide to prepare for reaming targeted depth of the posterior portion.

surface of the reaming guide (**Fig. 4**A). This distance is measured with a ruler (see **Fig. 4**B). If the distance is consistent from the superior to the inferior portion of the posterior glenoid, then the stabilizing pins and preparation guide are removed (see **Fig. 4**C). If the estimated depth of the step is not consistent throughout the prepared surface, additional rasping is performed until the surface is satisfactory. This step is important for assuring complete seating of the component and avoiding superior tilt of the glenoid component.

Bone Preparation Assessment and Tamping

After the posterior preparation guide has been removed, a final assessment of glenoid preparation is performed using a trial sizer disc of the appropriate glenoid size and step depth (see **Fig. 4**D). It is set onto the glenoid face, and the surgeon confirms that it does not rock, lift off, or wobble.

Drilling Peripheral Peg Holes

If the sizer disc fits well and is stable, the peripheral drill holes are made using the stepped peripheral

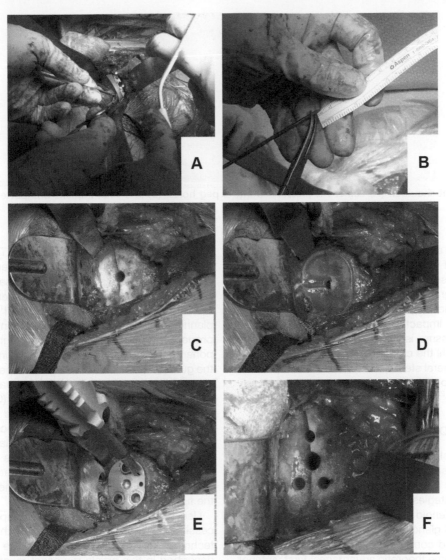

Fig. 4. Right shoulder. (*A*) The surgeon should put a free guide pin onto the posterior surface of the glenoid and clamp a Schnidt at the inferior surface of reaming guide. (*B*) The distance between the clamp and the tip is measured with a ruler. (*C*) The rasp guide is removed after the targeted reaming is completed. (*D*) The surgeon should determine whether the reamed glenoid surface is sufficient for accepting the implant by placing the appropriately sized bone preparation assessor. (*E*) The peripheral drill guide is inserted into the central hole. (*F*) The peripheral drill guide is removed. All 3 peripheral holes do not penetrate the cortical wall of the glenoid vault.

drill guide. The peripheral drill guide corresponding to the chosen step depth is inserted into the central hole, making sure it fully contacts the anteriorly and posteriorly prepared bony surface (see **Fig. 4**E). First, the anterior hole is drilled, followed by the posterior/inferior hole, and last, the superior hole. At the time of drilling, the author confirms whether the drill holes perforated the cortical wall of the glenoid vault (see **Fig. 4**F). The reason for this order is as follows: the superior hole spans the superior/inferior step in the glenoid bone and the posterior portion of the glenoid has already been removed. Hence, to prevent the peripheral

drill guide from shifting or rotating during the drilling of subsequent holes, the author prefers the order of drilling described above. If any of the peripheral drill holes have exited the glenoid vault, cancellous bone from the resected humeral head is inserted into the hole before placing the component trial.

Trialing/Final Implant

The glenoid trial is inserted and confirmed to fit appropriately. The trial is then removed, and holes are irrigated and dried. Any holes that had been

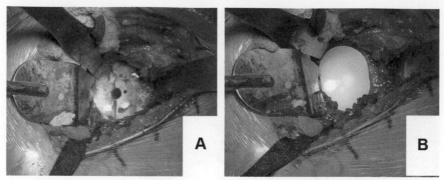

Fig. 5. Right shoulder. (*A*) Cement is pressurized into 3 peg holes. (*B*) The final implant is impacted onto the glenoid.

perforated and grafted are inspected to verify that the floor of the hole has been re-created. Cement is then pressurized into the peg holes (**Fig. 5**A) that were not grafted, and cement without pressurization is placed into any grafted holes. The final implant is impacted into position (see **Fig. 5**B). Direct pressure is maintained on the face of the implant until the cement hardens.

The humeral stem and head are then implanted, and the osteotomy is repaired as previously described.[25]

DISCUSSION

The optimal surgical treatment of posterior glenoid bone loss and increased retroversion is controversial. In this article, the author describes the treatment strategies for use of an augmented, stepped glenoid component to treat type B2 and selected C glenoids (ie, C2). Utilization of a stepped glenoid component in this setting has some real and some theoretic advantages. First, anterior glenoid bone can be preserved. Second, the lateral joint line is restored. Third, subchondral bone remains relatively preserved. Fourth, the size of the stepped component used can be individualized to the patient's specific anatomy. In addition, the stepped design may have biomechanically superior fixation and less anterior glenoid liftoff in the presence of eccentric glenoid bone loss when compared with other components, such as spherical asymmetric, spherical symmetric, flat angled, and anchor peg glenoid designs.[26] These perceived benefits may result in improved functional results and longer implant survival in this challenging treatment population. Youderian and colleagues[27] reported good to excellent clinical and structural results in 24 cases after shoulder arthroplasty using a stepped, posteriorly augmented glenoid component (Global Steptech APG, Depuy, Warsaw, IN, USA) at a

minimum of 6 months of follow-up. To validate the efficacy of augmented stepped glenoid components, long-term studies are necessary.

Despite these perceived benefits, there are also concerns. Surgeons require optimal operative planning and technique, especially in terms of proper sizing and determining the height of components. In addition, it can be challenging to place the guide pin in a location that avoids peg perforation. As aforementioned, the author has recently made use of image analysis software (Ortho Vis). There are multiple software options available, and there are likely to be more. The important point is that accurate glenoid component placement is difficult, especially in cases with severe deformity. It is likely that some type of preoperative/intraoperative planning system will be routinely used in the future.

Use of an augmented glenoid component necessitates a keen understanding of the surgical technique and its potential pitfalls. The strategies described in this article represent recently developed techniques that have not been studied with long-term clinical outcomes. Given the limitations associated with asymmetric reaming and bone grafting in the setting of B2 and C glenoids, augmented components may allow for improved outcomes for this difficult treatment population.

REFERENCES

1. Denard PJ, Walch G. Current concept in the surgical management of primary glenohumeral arthritis with a biconcave glenoid. J Shoulder Elbow Surg 2013; 22(11):1589–98.
2. Hsu J, Ricchetti ET, Huffman GR, et al. Addressing glenoid bone deficiency and asymmetric posterior erosion in shoulder arthroplasty. J Shoulder Elbow Surg 2013;22(12):1298–308.
3. Sears BW, Johnston PS, Ramsey ML, et al. Glenoid bone loss in primary total arthroplasty: evaluation

and management. J Am Acad Orthop Surg 2012; 20(9):604–13.

4. Walch G, Badet R, Boulahia A, et al. Morphologic study of the glenoid in primary glenohumeral osteoarthritis. J Arthroplasty 1999;14(6):756–60.

5. Sabesan V, Callanan M, Sharma V, et al. Correction of acquired glenoid bone loss in osteoarthritis with a standard versus an augmented glenoid component. J Shoulder Elbow Surg 2014;23(7):964–73.

6. Clavert P, Millett PJ, Warner JP. Glenoid resurfacing: what are the limits to asymmetric reaming for posterior erosion? J Shoulder Elbow Surg 2007;16(6): 843–8.

7. Gillespie R, Lyons R, Lazarus M. Eccentric reaming in total shoulder arthroplasty: a study. Orthopedics 2009;32(1):21.

8. Walch G, Young AA, Boileau P, et al. Patterns of loosening of polyethylene keeled glenoid components after shoulder arthroplasty for primary osteoarthritis: results of a multicenter study with more than five years of follow-up. J Bone Joint Surg Am 2012; 94(2):145–50.

9. Walch G, Moraga C, Young A, et al. Results of anatomic nonconstrained prosthesis in primary osteoarthritis with biconcave glenoid. J Shoulder Elbow Surg 2012;21(11):1526–33.

10. Gerber C, Costouros JG, Sukthankar A, et al. Static posterior humeral head subluxation and total shoulder arthroplasty. J Shoulder Elbow Surg 2009;18(4): 505–10.

11. Habermeyer P, Magosch P, Lichtenberg S. Recentering the humeral head for glenoid deficiency in total shoulder arthroplasty. Clin Orthop Relat Res 2007;457(4):124–32.

12. Clinton J, Franta AK, Lenters TR, et al. Nonprosthetic glenoid arthroplasty with humeral hemiarthroplasty and total shoulder arthroplasty yield similar self-assessed outcomes in the management of comparable patients with glenohumeral arthritis. J Shoulder Elbow Surg 2007;16(5):534–8.

13. Matsen FA 3rd, Gupta A. Axillary view: arthritic glenohumeral anatomy and changes after ream and run. Clin Orthop Relat Res 2014;472(3):894–902.

14. Gilmer BB, Comstock BA, Jette JL, et al. The prognosis for improvement in comfort and function after the ream-and-run arthroplasty for glenohumeral arthritis: an analysis of 176 consecutive cases. J Bone Joint Surg Am 2012;94(14):e102.

15. Neer CS II, Morrison DS. Glenoid bone-grafting in total shoulder arthroplasty. J Bone Joint Surg Am 1988;70(8):1154–62.

16. Steinmann SP, Cofield RH. Bone grafting for glenoid deficiency in total shoulder replacement. J Shoulder Elbow Surg 2000;9(5):361–7.

17. Hill JM, Norris TR. Long-term results of total shoulder arthroplasty following bone-grafting of the glenoid. J Bone Joint Surg Am 2001;83(6):877–83.

18. Sabesan V, Callanan M, Ho J, et al. Clinical and radiographic outcomes of total shoulder arthroplasty with bone graft for osteoarthritis with severe glenoid bone loss. J Bone Joint Surg Am 2013; 95(14):1290–6.

19. Iannotti JP, Greeson C, Downing D, et al. Effect of glenoid deformity on glenoid component placement in primary shoulder arthroplasty. J Shoulder Elbow Surg 2012;21(11):48–55.

20. Mizuno N, Denard PJ, Raiss P, et al. Reverse total shoulder arthroplasty for primary glenohumeral osteoarthritis in patients with a biconcave glenoid. J Bone Joint Surg Am 2013;95(14):1297–304.

21. Bonnevialle N, Mansat P, Mansat M, et al. Hemiarthroplasty for osteoarthritis in shoulder with dysplastic morphology. J Shoulder Elbow Surg 2011; 20(3):378–84.

22. Edwards TB, Boulahia A, Kempf JF, et al. Shoulder arthroplasty in osteoarthritis and dysplastic glenoid morphology. J Shoulder Elbow Surg 2004;13(1):1–4.

23. Sperling JW, Cofield RH, Steinmann SP. Shoulder arthroplasty for osteoarthritis secondary to glenoid dysplasia. J Bone Joint Surg Am 2002;84(4):541–6.

24. Gunther SB, Lynch TL. Total shoulder replacement surgery with custom glenoid implants for severe bone deficiency. J Shoulder Elbow Surg 2012; 21(5):675–84.

25. Williams GR, Ramsey ML. Hemiarthroplasty, total shoulder arthroplasty, and biologic glenoid resurfacing for glenohumeral arthritis with an intact rotator cuff. In: Wiesel SW, editor. Operative techniques in shoulder and elbow surgery. Philadelphia: Lipppincott Williams and Wilkins; 2010. p. 220–33.

26. Iannotti JP, Lappin KE, Klotz CL, et al. Liftoff resistance of augmented glenoid components during cyclic fatigue loading in the posterior-superior direction. J Shoulder Elbow Surg 2013;22(11):1530–6.

27. Youderian AR, Napolitano LA, Davidson IU, et al. Management of glenoid bone loss with the use of a new augmented all-polyethylene glenoid component. Technique in Shoulder and Elbow Surgery 2012;13(4):163–9.

Pain Management Strategies in Hand Surgery

Constantinos Ketonis, MD, PhD*, Asif M. Ilyas, MD,
Frederic Liss, MD

KEYWORDS

- Ambulatory hand surgery • Wide-awake surgery • Combination analgesics • Nerve block • Exparel

KEY POINTS

- The choice of intraoperative anesthesia and a postoperative oral pain medication regiment can have a great effect on the patients' hospital length of stay and recovery experience.
- General anesthesia and regional or local blocks with sedation continue to provide safe, effective perioperative anesthesia and, therefore, have maintained a strong presence in hand surgery.
- Wide-awake hand surgery can be used for a growing number of hand procedures and can avoid the need and cost for preoperative testing and potentially decreases postoperative complications and narcotic consumption.
- New Bier block modifications, including more distal tourniquet placement, allow for the use of less anesthetic making it a safer and more efficient technique.
- There is a shift away from opioid analgesic monotherapies toward combination formulations with complementary mechanisms of oral agents that can achieve greater efficacy and safety profile.
- Bupivacaine liposome formulation has been approved for single-shot surgical wound infiltration and can theoretically lead to pain relief for up to 96 hours postoperatively.

INTRODUCTION

The growth in both medical technology and the availability of better anesthetic agents has triggered a dramatic growth in ambulatory surgery over the last 2 decades. The rapid onset and termination of effect of modern anesthetic agents as well as a better understanding of their mechanism of action has allowed longer cases to be performed on an ambulatory basis with quicker recovery of patients allowing safe same-day discharge to home.[1] As of 2003, 70% of the surgical procedures in North America were performed on an ambulatory basis, and it now accounts for most surgeries performed in the United States, some European countries, and Australia.[1,2] Orthopedic surgery, and in particular hand surgical procedures, account for a large portion of these outpatient surgeries[3] and are likely only to increase with time as economic restrictions continue to influence the way we practice. Leblanc and colleagues[4] analyzed the cost and efficiency associated with performing carpal tunnel releases in the main operating room as compared with the ambulatory setting and found that the use of the main operating room for carpal tunnel releases is almost 4 times as expensive and less than half as efficient as when performed in an ambulatory setting.

Disclosures: No animals or human subjects were involved in the production of this article.

The authors of this study have no conflicts of interest.

Rothman Institute at Thomas Jefferson University Hospital, 925 Chestnut Street, 5th Floor, Philadelphia, PA 19107, USA

* Corresponding author. Rothman Institute, Tissue Engineering & Regenerative Medicine/Department of Orthopaedic Surgery, Thomas Jefferson University Hospital, 1015 Walnut Street, Suite 501, Philadelphia, PA 19107.

E-mail address: ketonis@gmail.com

Orthop Clin N Am 46 (2015) 399–408
http://dx.doi.org/10.1016/j.ocl.2015.02.008

Even though expense and efficiency are important driving factors, perhaps the main prerequisite for performing ambulatory surgery is postoperative pain that can be controlled with oral analgesics. With the ever-expanding boundaries of what can be done as an outpatient, safe and effective pain control remains an important challenge for surgeons and patients alike.[5] It is estimated that up to 30% to 40% of ambulatory surgical patients suffer from moderate to severe pain during the first 24 to 48 hours after their discharge,[2] which often times will interfere with sleep and daily functioning. Even though this improves with time, postoperative pain remains the most common reason for recurrent office visits and unanticipated hospital admission.[6–8] Chung and colleagues[3] prospectively studied 1008 consecutive ambulatory surgical patients across 8 surgical specialties and found that in the recovery room or postanesthesia care units (PACUs), orthopedic patients (including hand surgical procedures) had the highest incidence of pain, more than urologic, general surgery, and plastic surgery patients. Furthermore, in a survey by Rawal and colleagues[7] that analyzed postoperative pain, it was found that 37% of hand surgery patients will have moderate to severe pain postoperatively, affecting their function and quality of life.

Traditionally the patient's pain is managed with general anesthesia (GA) and narcotic medication for surgery, followed by oral medications, including acetaminophen, nonsteroidal antiinflammatory drugs (NSAIDs), opioid-containing oral analgesics (eg, codeine-acetaminophen), or a combination of these.[9] Despite the availability of these analgesic drugs, many patients still do not achieve adequate pain control,[10] often times because adverse gastrointestinal, hemostatic, and renal effects become prohibitive to achieving adequate analgesic concentrations.

INTRAOPERATIVE ANALGESIA

The choice of analgesia and anesthesia during the surgical procedure can have a great effect on the pain level and chance of successful pain control postoperatively and often dictates both the extent of preoperative evaluation and the postoperative length of stay of patients in the hospital after the procedure. The techniques that are discussed here include GA, peripheral nerve blocks, intravenous (IV) regional blocks, and local anesthesia with or without sedation.

General Anesthesia

GA has a long established history and safe profile. It involves complete anesthetization of patients requiring intubation and artificial ventilation. It has been previously established in the shoulder literature[11,12] that GA, as compared with peripheral regional blocks (PRBs), results in longer recovery times and slower hospital discharge after surgery. Similarly, Chan and colleagues[13] prospectively examined 3 anesthetic techniques during hand surgical procedures, specifically GA, peripheral (axillary) regional block, and IV regional anesthesia (IVRA), with respect to clinical outcome, time efficiency, and hospital cost. They found that regional anesthesia is associated with a more favorable patient recovery profile than GA, requiring less nursing care in the recovery room and an earlier hospital discharge. These findings were redemonstrated later by McCartney and colleagues[14] in a prospective randomized trial of 100 ambulatory hand surgery patients demonstrating that single-shot axillary PRB significantly reduces pain in the immediate postoperative period, reducing recovery room times and total hospital time and increasing the time to the first analgesic request before discharge. However, when they tracked patient-reported pain beyond the immediate postoperative period, they found no difference in pain level on postoperative day 1 or up to 14 days after surgery when compared with GA.

Peripheral Regional Blocks

Single-injection plexus blocks are currently the most commonly used modality for PRBs in upper extremity surgery. First performed by the American surgeon William Stuart Halsted in 1885, it involves injecting a local anesthetic in the area of the brachial plexus, which can provide analgesic effects from 12 to 24 hours.[15,16] Depending on the surgical area, this can be administered as an interscalene, supraclavicular, or infraclavicular block. The most common block is the interscalene block that affects the root-trunk level of the brachial plexus and can be used for procedures involving the shoulder, proximal aspect of the humerus, and distal aspect of the clavicle but is inadequate for procedures that are distal to the elbow. The supraclavicular block, that affects the anterior and posterior divisions of the trunks of the brachial plexus, as well as the infraclavicular nerve block that targets the brachial plexus at the level of the cords before the exit of the axillary and musculocutaneous nerves, is well suited for procedures involving the arm, elbow, forearm, and hand. Finally, the suprascapular and axillary nerve blocks have a similar coverage with the interscalene block, and can be an effective option for intraoperative and postoperative pain control for shoulder procedures.

Overall, PRBs can offer cost-effective pain control for patients undergoing upper extremity procedures and have the potential to minimize the need for postoperative narcotic use, shorter hospital stays, and increased patient satisfaction.[9] Nevertheless, several complications have been reported with the use of these blocks, including pneumothorax, recurrent laryngeal nerve blockade, phrenic blockade, peripheral neuropathy, spinal cord damage, and sympathetic chain blockade.[17] With the use of ultrasound guidance, the safety of PRBs has been enhanced and allows for more accurate placement of the blocks with lower anesthetic volumes.

Intravenous Regional Anesthesia

IVRA, more readily known as the Bier block, was first developed by Dr August Bier in 1908 and still remains an effective regional anesthesia technique frequently used for upper extremity surgery. It generally involves placement of a tourniquet above the elbow, exsanguination of the extremity with an Esmarch and tourniquet inflation to ensure arterial occlusion, followed by slow injection of an anesthetic agent (typically lidocaine) into the IV cannula of the surgical hand.[18]

The Bier block technique is intended to provide a bloodless field with rapid onset and high reliability of complete anesthesia, eliminating the need for GA, all while leaving local tissue or anatomic structures undistorted.[19] However, this technique is often associated with tourniquet pain and, therefore, may still require sedation for patient comfort,[20] which is associated with all the well-described side effects of nausea, vomiting, and decreased cognitive function. These side effects, along with failure to provide adequate postoperative analgesia,[21] ultimately impact the time to discharge. In an effort to improve the quality of the block, over the years, various adjuvants have been added to the local anesthetic solution, including opioids, NSAIDs, (alpha)$_2$-adrenergic agonists, sodium bicarbonate, and muscle relaxants,[21] with varying degrees of success.

Another concern associated with the Bier block is its potential to cause both local and systemic pharmacologic toxicity as the tourniquet is deflated, and various serious complications including death have been reported in the literature.[18–24] Guay[22] recently performed a systematic review of the adverse events associated with Bier blocks and described cases of local anesthetic toxicity, compartment syndrome, cardiac arrests, and deaths, as well as seizures that have been reported even with lidocaine at its lowest effective dose (1.5 mg/kg). He concluded that even though serious complications might result from the utilization of the Bier block, their incidence is relatively low; therefore, this technique can be considered a safe method of providing anesthesia during surgery. To minimize these risks, precautionary measures have been described when using this technique. To reduce the bolus effect of the anesthetic agent as it is released into the general circulation,[19] cyclical release of the tourniquet is most times necessary. Additionally, a minimum tourniquet time of 30 minutes is required when using a Bier block,[23] ensuring enough diffusion of the total anesthetic agent before allowing its systemic distribution. This time limitation may make the use of the Bier block impractical for shorter procedures further narrowing its indications in outpatient hand procedures.

In recent years, there has been a renewed interest in reviving and enhancing Bier blocks. Investigators have described modifications to the Bier block technique, such as placing the tourniquet distal to the elbow thereby reducing the amount of lidocaine used to achieve adequate anesthesia and also decreasing the amount of time the tourniquet must remain inflated. Arslanian and colleagues[23] described their experience with forearm Bier block in 121 procedures performed and interviewed patients by telephone 24 hours postoperatively. They report that all patients received adequate anesthesia from the block with no intraoperative or postoperative complications. They were also able to reduce the tourniquet time to about 10.1 minutes using this technique.

Another area of adjustment has been in the choice of anesthetic agent. Mepivacaine, prilocaine, and bupivacaine[24] or the use of adjunctive analgesics, such as ketorolac and combinations thereof,[25] have been described in the literature to provide varying durations of action and blockade. Opioids, including morphine,[26] fentanyl[27] sufentanil, and meperidine, have been added to the Bier block solution with contradictory results.[28] Nonetheless, lidocaine, which is typically given as 0.5% plain lidocaine at a maximum dose of 3 mg/kg, still remains one of the more common anesthetics used for Bier blocks because of its low potential for systemic toxicity.

Wide-Awake Surgery

Wide-awake hand surgery was first introduced by Lalonde about a decade ago,[29,30] which he termed wide awake local anesthesia no tourniquet (WA-LANT). It involves injecting a local anesthetic with epinephrine directly into the surgical field without sedation or a tourniquet. Patients are entirely awake. In order to minimize injection discomfort, Lalonde recommends adding bicarbonate to the anesthetic in order to normalize the pH as well as slowly delivering it in a controlled manner using a 27-g or smaller needle.

Epinephrine is a potent vasoconstrictor, which decreases the bleeding in the surgical field, thus, avoiding the need for a tourniquet that is known to cause considerable discomfort, which alone often warrants sedation. This idea became possible after the emergence of recent evidence suggesting that it is safe to inject epinephrine in the human finger, previously thought to potentially lead to digital ischemia and necrosis.[31,32] Subsequently, negating the need for the tourniquet avoids the need for sedation. Furthermore, lidocaine provides the local anesthesia allowing patients to undergo both simple operations, such as carpal tunnel releases and Dupuytren excisions, as well as more complex surgeries, such as arthroplasties[33] and tendon transfers[34], circumventing the need for GA, PRB, IVRA, or sedation and, hence, all the risks associated with them. In fact, Lalonde recently claimed that WALANT can be used for up to 95% of all hand surgery procedures.[35,36] Additional advantages of WALANT include significant cost savings as it forgoes the need for anesthesia, eliminates preoperative history and physicals, and preoperative diagnostic studies, such as blood work.[37–39] Furthermore, the ability to avoid anesthesia allows patients with significant comorbidities that would otherwise be denied surgery because of the risk of anesthesia to safely undergo hand surgical procedures. An added benefit is that because patients are awake during the procedures, they can receive education about their surgery and postoperative management and can also actively participate in the surgery by actively flexing and extending the digits so the surgeon can evaluate, for example, whether a tendon repair glides freely intraoperatively.

Elimination of anesthesia also means that patients can practically get up after surgery and go home with no need for extensive PACU care, medication administration, and the associated side effects, such as drowsiness, nausea, or vomiting. In a prospective cohort study by Davison and colleagues[40] that compared 100 consecutive carpal tunnel releases (CTR) done with only WALANT with 100 consecutive CTRs done with sedation, they found that 93% of the patients in either group would choose the same method of anesthesia they received again, demonstrating that people would choose the method that they are more familiar with. More importantly, they found that WALANT patients spent less time at the hospital than sedated patients (2.6 hours vs 4.0 hours, respectively) and that only 3% of WALANT patients required preoperative testing (blood work,

electrocardiograms, and/or chest radiographs) as compared with 48% of sedated patients. Additionally, preoperative anxiety levels for WALANT patients were lower than for sedated patients even though postoperative anxiety was similar. Narcotics were used by only 5% of unsedated patients as opposed to 67% of sedated patients despite reported adequate pain control by 89% and 90% of patients, respectively. Surprisingly, the postoperative nausea and vomiting incidence was very low for both groups in this study (1% and 7%), unlike most other previous studies.[41]

POSTOPERATIVE ANALGESIA
Postanesthesia Care Unit

Effective pain management in the PACU can have a big impact on patient satisfaction, time to discharge, and their postoperative experience once patients go home. Morphine and fentanyl are widely used in ambulatory patients to provide analgesia during phase I recovery. Fentanyl has been advocated because of its faster onset time and, therefore, more rapid pain control, potentially avoiding total opioid dose and related side effects. Claxton and colleagues[42] compared the use of IV morphine and fentanyl after painful ambulatory procedures in a prospective randomized trial and demonstrated that morphine produced a better quality of analgesia but was associated with an increased incidence of nausea and vomiting, most of which occurred after discharge. They concluded that the reduced side effects in combination with a short duration of action with fentanyl may facilitate earlier discharge and produce fewer complications after discharge.

Home Analgesia

Oral analgesia is the mainstay of pain control once patients leave the hospital. Medications prescribed should allow patients to perform normal activities of daily living, produce minimal side effects, not interfere with the healing process, and be easy to manage by patients. Depending on the type of procedure performed, breakthrough pain medications might also be indicated to keep pain under control in case the prescribed analgesic is ineffective. Postoperative pain after ambulatory hand surgery is typically managed with a combination of oral medications, including acetaminophen, NSAIDs, and opioid-containing oral analgesics (eg, codeine-acetaminophen). Regardless of the choice of medication, patient education on what to expect, ways to manage pain, and how to use the medications prescribed remains paramount.

Acetaminophen

Acetaminophen is one of the most widely used analgesics worldwide. It is effective, safe, inexpensive, and has a favorable adverse effect profile.[43] Yet, its mechanism of action is poorly understood. There is some evidence that it has a central antinociceptive effect, and some of the proposed mechanisms of action include inhibition of cyclooxygenase-2 (COX-2) or inhibition of putative central COX (COX-3).[44,45] There is also some evidence that it modulates inhibitory serotonergic pathways and may also prevent prostaglandin production at the cellular level. However, it is known that, unlike NSAIDs, acetaminophen does not irritate gastric mucosa, affect platelet function, or cause renal insufficiency, making it a very versatile medication.

Nonsteroidal antiinflammatory drugs

Prostaglandins, and their role in pain modulation, were first discovered in the 1960s. In 1965, Sir John Vane first demonstrated the in vivo reduction in prostaglandin levels by inhibition of prostaglandin synthetase, now known as COX.[46] Once this enzyme was identified, NSAIDs were developed to inhibit it. Even though some central action has been reported,[47] the generally accepted mechanism of action of NSAIDs today remains the attenuation of prostaglandin synthesis by inhibition of COX enzymes.[48]

NSAIDs are now part of most outpatient surgery pain regimens. Their antiinflammatory properties not only provide pain relief but may also help reduce local edema and minimize the use of more potent medications. The 1998 guidelines for the use of NSAIDs in the perioperative period, issued by the Royal College of Anesthetists, stated that based on the strongest evidence available, "in situations where there are no contraindications, NSAIDs are the drug of choice after many day-case procedures."[7] Today it is estimated that 20% to 30% of Americans use an NSAID each year, and 1% to 2% use NSAIDs every day.[49]

Despite their success, one of the main concerns with the use of NSAIDs remains their gastrointestinal toxicity, which led to the exploration of ways to reduce their side-effect profile. The two COX isoenzymes were discovered in the late 1980s, with COX-1 largely involved in homeostasis, including the maintenance of gastroprotective mechanisms and renal blood flow, and COX-2, which is upregulated during the inflammatory response. COX-2–selective drugs emerged shortly after the discovery of the isoenzymes, which the World Health Organization has categorized as a new subclass of NSAIDs (coxibs). Despite continuing controversy over the safety of the coxibs with concerns of a higher risk of myocardial infarction, there seems to be no clear differences in the cardiovascular risks of the currently available coxibs and the nonselective NSAIDs when used at the recommended doses.[46] On the other hand, even with a favorable side-effect profile, they perform equally as well as the nonselective NSAIDs. In a recent systematic review by Rømsing and Møiniche,[50] they showed that rofecoxib 50 mg and parecoxib 40 mg have an equipotent analgesic efficacy relative to traditional NSAIDs in postoperative pain after minor and major surgical procedures.

Ketorolac

Ketorolac is a newer NSAID analgesic, considered a central nervous system agent,[51] that was first approved for use by the US Food and Drug Administration (FDA) in 1997. Similar to classic nonselective NSAIDs, when coadministered with an opioid, it exhibits marked opioid-sparing effects, allowing a 25% to 50% reduction in opioid requirement.[51] A randomized double-blinded study by Kinsella and colleagues[52] demonstrated that morphine requirements were 3 times less in the first 24 hours in patients having major orthopedic procedures who had adjuvant ketorolac administered during the postoperative period.

Because it acts by inhibiting the COX pathway, it is, therefore, also a potent inhibitor of platelet aggregation; some concerns were raised with its use in the perioperative period for bleeding. Even though there is a paucity of literature in the use of ketorolac with hand surgical procedures in particular, it has been examined in the spine literature by Chin and colleagues,[53] who found no risk of bleeding complications compared with that of their control group in patients having microdiscectomy after a single intraoperative dose of ketorolac.

For all NSAIDs, careful patient selection is important. Specifically, a history of coronary artery disease, gastrointestinal risk factors such as gastric ulcers, and renal insufficiency has to be taken into consideration before prescribing nonselective NSAIDs, COX-2 selective inhibitors, or ketorolac. After weighing the risks and benefits, NSAIDs, when used at the right dose, remain one of the most effective analgesics and antiinflammatory medications that can safely be used for postoperative analgesia after hand surgical procedures.

Opioids

Even though opioids are routinely used in outpatient surgery in the United States, their role is sometimes questioned because of their well-known side effects of nausea, vomiting, sedation, dizziness, and respiratory depression and the risk of substance dependence.[54] Weak opioids, such as codeine and tramadol, are commonly used and are often times prescribed in combination with acetaminophen. In a controlled trial,[55] postoperative pain management at home using tramadol, metamizole, or acetaminophen as single substances after outpatient hand surgery has been shown to be inadequate for up to 40% of all patients. Consequently, there has been an increasing focus on combining analgesic medications with different mechanisms of action and complementary pharmacokinetic profiles in hopes to not only achieve greater efficacy but also a better safety profile.[56] For example, in a randomized, double-blind, multicenter trial comparing the efficacy and safety of tramadol 37.5 mg/acetaminophen 325-mg combination tablet compared with tramadol hydrochloride (HCL) 50 mg alone in the treatment of postoperative pain following outpatient hand surgery, it was found that analgesic efficacy of the 2 treatments was comparable; but the tramadol/acetaminophen treatment showed a better safety profile than the tramadol monotherapy.[57]

FUTURE DIRECTIONS

Extended, complete, and safe pain relief without the need for oral medication and minimal effort from patients are the desired characteristics of an ideal analgesic strategy. Oral or IV analgesics are by definition systemic medications and invariably are associated with side effects. One also has to consider possible medication interactions, use of concurrent anticoagulation treatment, and any preexisting conditions or comorbidities as these can affect the clearance and effective dosing of the analgesic used. A local or peripheral analgesic strategy can minimize the need for systemic medications and can potentially not only decrease the risks of associated side effects as well as potential medication interactions but also relies less on patient compliance and requires less customization from patient to patient.

Continuous Peripheral Nerve Blockade

The strategy of continuous peripheral nerve blockade (CPNB) for postoperative analgesia entails the percutaneous insertion of perineural catheters close to the peripheral nerve of interest and the continuous infusion of local anesthetic to achieve blockade in its corresponding distribution. Richman and colleagues[54] conducted a meta-analysis of randomized controlled studies comparing the effectiveness of CPNB and opioids. They identified 19 studies (12 of which for upper extremity procedures) including more than 600 patients and revealed that CPNB provided better

postoperative analgesia compared with opioids at 24 hours, 48 hours, and 72 hours postoperatively. Furthermore, a significant reduction in opioid use (when used as a rescue medication) was noted in patients receiving perineural analgesia with fewer opioid-related side effects.

However, variable success rates of CNPB have been reported in the literature. In a single-center, prospective, double-blind, randomized, and placebo-controlled study, Goebel and colleagues[58] compared single-shot and CPNB by insertion of a patient-controlled interscalene catheter, using 0.2% ropivacaine, after major open-shoulder surgeries that showed significantly less consumption of rescue medication in the catheter group but only within the first 24 hours after surgery; opioid use past day 1 was equal in the 2 groups, with no differences in the incidence of side effects.

Catheter patency or secondary catheter block has been identified in many studies as a major mode of failure of CPNB with rates ranging from 10% to 20%.[59–61] Even though most studies have been limited by small patient samples, one of the largest series ever published, comes from the hand literature. Ahsan and colleagues[62] retrospectively explored the incidence of failure in 207 patients who received infraclavicular or supraclavicular CPNB for postoperative analgesia after upper extremity surgery. In their series, the CPNB failure rate for infraclavicular and supraclavicular catheters was 19% and 26%, respectively. Other mechanisms of CNPB failure that have been reported and could explain these results include catheter migration,[63] fluid leakage at the catheter site,[59] and dislodgement or obstruction of the tubing.[64] Incorrect catheter placement,[65] despite the significant increase in placement accuracy with the use of ultrasound guidance, also still remains an issue.

In addition to the failures associated with the pump, catheter, and block placement, serious complications related to the the use of CPNB as an analgesic technique in general have been reported, such as peri-catheter hematoma formation and intravascular puncture,[66] myonecrosis, systemic or local anesthetic toxicity, and prolonged Horner syndrome.[67] The presence of a catheter that violates the skin also raises the concern for introduction of bacteria to the area, and infection rates after catheter placement have been reported to be 0% to 3%.[68]

Furthermore, their satisfactory function relies on patients taking care of the pump at home. In order to implement these systems in the ambulatory setting, one must assure that the patients are well educated on how to care for them and make sure there is very stringent follow-up in place.

Extended Local Blocks

Multiple attempts have been made to extend the effect of local anesthetics and blocks to attain longer local and regional anesthesia in the early postoperative period thereby decreasing the need for both narcotics and NSAIDs. Despite multiple efforts and approaches with the use of adjuvants, vehicles, and gel formulations of classic analgesics and anesthetics, the typical duration of adequate pain control has been a maximum of 24 hours.

Recently an extended-acting local anesthetic in the form of bupivacaine liposome has been introduced. The agent is commercially known as Exparel and was granted FDA approval in 2011,[69] as a local single-shot injection into the surgical site for postsurgical pain relief. The extended-release formulation consists of microscopic, spherical lipids, which allow for diffusion of bupivacaine over an extended period, resulting in pain relief for up to 96 hours after surgery. In contrast, infiltration with classic local anesthetic agents that are widely used today, result in analgesia that is generally limited to less than 24 hours.

In a recent randomized, multicenter, double-blind, phase 3 clinical study,[70] Exparel was compared with placebo for the prevention of pain after bunionectomy. Using a numeric rating scale for pain, scores were significantly less in patients treated with Exparel as compared with patients receiving placebo at 24 and 36 hours. They also found that more patients in the Exparel group avoided use of opioid rescue medication during the first 24 hours and were pain free up to 48 hours after surgery. Moreover, fewer adverse events were reported by patients treated with Exparel (59.8%) versus placebo (67.7%). Similarly, Portillo and colleagues[71] completed a systematic review of prospective studies on the use of Exparel in various surgeries, including knee arthroplasty, hemorrhoidectomy, augmentation mammoplasty, and bunionectomy and found that Exparel was well tolerated and showed a favorable safety profile compared with the controls.

To the best of the authors' knowledge, no studies have been conducted to date that explore the use of Exparel specifically in hand surgery. Such studies are needed to validate the use of this agent in these procedures.

Extended Peripheral Nerve Blocks

Currently available local anesthetics approved for single-injection peripheral nerve blocks have a maximum duration of less than 24 hours. Just as in the case of extended local blocks, attempts have been made to prolong the duration of peripheral nerve blocks with the use of various vehicles, such as implantable pellets,[72] hyaluronic acid matrices,[73] or lipid-protein-sugar particles,[74] just to name a few. However, clinical translation and wide adoption of such systems of sustained-release formulations for local anesthetics has mostly been limited by adverse tissue reaction with reports of myotoxicity, inflammation, and neurotoxicity.

Exparel, which is known to release for up to 96 hours after injection, is currently FDA approved exclusively for local surgical site infiltration but not for peripheral nerve blocks.[75] Studies on the use of Exparel in peripheral nerve blockade are beginning to emerge. In plastic surgery, Morales and colleagues[76] report their experience with 64 female patients who received Exparel injections in an abdominal field block fashion for abdominoplasty with rectus plication. Based on their postoperative data and questionnaires, these patients experienced reduced postoperative pain, required less postoperative narcotic medication, and resumed both earlier ambulation and normal activity. Furthermore, Ilfeld and colleagues[75] administered bilateral single-injection Exparel femoral nerve blocks in 14 healthy volunteers. Using the maximum voluntary isometric contraction of the quadriceps femoris muscle and tolerance to cutaneous electrical current in the femoral nerve distribution as end points, they reported partial sensory and motor block of greater than 24 hours.

Exparel's biocompatibility near nerve tissue is not well characterized, but a few studies have began to look at the safety in such scenarios. McAlvin and colleagues[77] injected Exparel close to the sciatic nerves in rats and compared its effects with that of different concentrations of bupivacaine HCL. They found that even though Exparel injection caused a longer sciatic nerve blockade, median inflammation scores determined by histologic sections 4 days after injection were slightly higher. However, myotoxicity in all groups was not statistically different and no neurotoxicity was detected in any group. Richard and colleagues[78] performed single-dose toxicology studies of 3 doses of Exparel (9, 18, and 30 mg/kg) and compared them with bupivacaine (9 mg/kg) and saline. When these were injected around the brachial plexus nerve bundle of rabbits and dogs, they found that at the same dose, Exparel resulted in a 4-fold lower maximum plasma concentration of bupivacaine and was well tolerated at all doses. Histopathology evaluation on days 3 and 15 only revealed minimal to mild granulomatous inflammation of adipose tissue around nerve roots and concluded that it did not produce any nerve damage in their model.

Exparel continues to be actively investigated for postsurgical analgesia via peripheral nerve block,[78] and so far two phase 1 studies have been completed. Based on the safety data, the FDA has now approved subsequent phase 2 and 3 trials. If this, along with other newer analgesics, continues to prove safe and efficacious, we may soon be able to provide long-lasting pain relief to patients undergoing ambulatory hand procedures without the use of oral medications and, hence, without their well described side effects.

REFERENCES

1. Pregler JL, Kapur PA. The development of ambulatory anesthesia and future challenges. Anesthesiol Clin North America 2003;21(2):207–28.
2. Rawal N. Postoperative pain treatment for ambulatory surgery. Best Pract Res Clin Anaesthesiol 2007;21(1):129–48.
3. Chung F, Ritchie E, Su J. Postoperative pain in ambulatory surgery. Anesth Analg 1997;85(4):808–16.
4. Leblanc MR, Lalonde J, Lalonde DH. A detailed cost and efficiency analysis of performing carpal tunnel surgery in the main operating room versus the ambulatory setting in Canada. Hand (N Y) 2007; 2(4):173–8.
5. Meridy HW. Criteria for selection of ambulatory surgical patients and guidelines for anesthetic management: a retrospective study of 1553 cases. Anesth Analg 1982;61(11):921–6.
6. Beauregard L, Pomp A, Choinière M. Severity and impact of pain after day-surgery. Can J Anaesth 1998;45(4):304–11.
7. Rawal N, Hylander J, Nydahl PA, et al. Survey of postoperative analgesia following ambulatory surgery. Acta Anaesthesiol Scand 1997;41(8): 1017–22.
8. Wu CL, Berenholtz SM, Pronovost PJ, et al. Systematic review and analysis of postdischarge symptoms after outpatient surgery. Anesthesiology 2002;96(4): 994–1003.
9. Srikumaran U, Stein BE, Tan EW, et al. Upper-extremity peripheral nerve blocks in the perioperative pain management of orthopaedic patients: AAOS exhibit selection. J Bone Joint Surg Am 2013; 95(24). e197(1–13).
10. Dolin SJ, Cashman JN, Bland JM. Effectiveness of acute postoperative pain management: I. Evidence from published data. Br J Anaesth 2002;89(3): 409–23.
11. D'Alessio JG, Rosenblum M, Shea KP, et al. A retrospective comparison of interscalene block and general anesthesia for ambulatory surgery shoulder arthroscopy. Reg Anesth 1995;20(1):62–8.
12. Brown AR, Weiss R, Greenberg C, et al. Interscalene block for shoulder arthroscopy: comparison with general anesthesia. Arthroscopy 1993;9(3):295–300.
13. Chan VW, Peng PW, Kaszas Z, et al. A comparative study of general anesthesia, intravenous regional anesthesia, and axillary block for outpatient hand surgery: clinical outcome and cost analysis. Anesth Analg 2001;93(5):1181–4.
14. McCartney CJ, Brull R, Chan VW, et al. Early but no long-term benefit of regional compared with general anesthesia for ambulatory hand surgery. Anesthesiology 2004;101(2):461–7.
15. Gohl MR, Moeller RK, Olson RL, et al. The addition of interscalene block to general anesthesia for patients undergoing open shoulder procedures. AANA J 2001;69(2):105–9.
16. Kinnard P, Truchon R, St-Pierre A, et al. Interscalene block for pain relief after shoulder surgery. A prospective randomized study. Clin Orthop Relat Res 1994;(304):22–4.
17. Russon K, Pickworth T, Harrop-Griffiths W. Upper limb blocks. Anaesthesia 2010;65(Suppl 1):48–56.
18. Brill S, Middleton W, Brill G, et al. Bier's block; 100 years old and still going strong! Acta Anaesthesiol Scand 2004;48(1):117–22. Available at: http://onlinelibrary. wiley.com/doi/10.1111/j.1399-6576.2004.00280.x/full.
19. Colbern E. The Bier block for intravenous regional anesthesia: technic and literature review. Anesth Analg 1970;49(6):935–40.
20. Chiao FB, Chen J, Lesser JB, et al. Single-cuff forearm tourniquet in intravenous regional anaesthesia results in less pain and fewer sedation requirements than upper arm tourniquet. Br J Anaesth 2013; 111(2):271–5.
21. Joshi GP. Recent developments in regional anesthesia for ambulatory surgery. Curr Opin Anaesthesiol 1999;12(6):643–7.
22. Guay J. Adverse events associated with intravenous regional anesthesia (Bier block): a systematic review of complications. J Clin Anesth 2009;21(8):585–94. Available at: http://linkinghub.elsevier.com/retrieve/ pii/S0952818009002827.
23. Arslanian B, Mehrzad R, Kramer T, et al. Forearm Bier block: a new regional anesthetic technique for upper extremity surgery. Ann Plast Surg 2014; 73(2):156–7.
24. Pickering SA, Hunter JB. Bier's block using prilocaine: safe, cheap and well tolerated. Surgeon 2003;1(5):283–5.
25. Singh R, Bhagwat A, Bhadoria P, et al. Forearm IVRA, using 0.5% lidocaine in a dose of 1.5 mg/kg with ketorolac 0.15 mg/kg for hand and wrist surgeries. Minerva Anestesiol 2010;76(2):109–14.
26. Gupta A, Björnsson A, Sjöberg F, et al. Lack of peripheral analgesic effect of low-dose morphine during intravenous regional anesthesia. Reg Anesth 1993;18(4):250–3.

27. Armstrong P, Power I, Wildsmith JA. Addition of fentanyl to prilocaine for intravenous regional anaesthesia. Anaesthesia 1991;46(4):278–80.

28. Reuben SS, Steinberg RB, Klatt JL, et al. Intravenous regional anesthesia using lidocaine and clonidine. Anesthesiology 1999;91(3):654–8.

29. Thomson CJ, Lalonde DH, Denkler KA, et al. A critical look at the evidence for and against elective epinephrine use in the finger. Plast Reconstr Surg 2007;119(1):260–6.

30. Lalonde DH, Bell M, Benoit P, et al. A Multicenter Prospective Study of 3,110 Consecutive Cases of Elective Epinephrine Use in the Fingers and Hand: The Dalhousie Project Clinical Phase. J Hand Surg Am 2005;30(5):1061–7.

31. Krunic AL, Wang LC, Soltani K, et al. Digital anesthesia with epinephrine: an old myth revisited. J Am Acad Dermatol 2004;51(5):755–9.

32. Denkler K. A comprehensive review of epinephrine in the finger: to do or not to do. Plast Reconstr Surg 2001;108(1):114–24.

33. Farhangkhoee H, Lalonde J, Lalonde DH. Wide-awake trapeziectomy: video detailing local anesthetic injection and surgery. Hand (N Y) 2011;6(4):466–7.

34. Bezuhly M, Sparkes GL, Higgins A, et al. Immediate thumb extension following extensor indicis proprius-to-extensor pollicis longus tendon transfer using the wide-awake approach. Plast Reconstr Surg 2007; 119(5):1507–12.

35. Lalonde DH. How the wide awake approach is changing hand surgery and hand therapy: inaugural AAHS sponsored lecture at the ASHT meeting, San Diego, 2012. J Hand Ther 2013;26(2):175–8. Available at: http://eutils.ncbi.nlm.nih.gov/entrez/eutils/e link.fcgi?dbfrom=pubmed&id=23294825&retmode =ref&cmd=prlinks.

36. Lalonde DH, Wong A. Dosage of local anesthesia in wide awake hand surgery. J Hand Surg Am 2013; 38(10):2025–8.

37. Bismil M, Bismil Q, Harding D, et al. Transition to total one-stop wide-awake hand surgery service-audit: a retrospective review. JRSM Short Rep 2012;3(4):23.

38. Lalonde DH. Reconstruction of the hand with wide awake surgery. Clin Plast Surg 2011;38(4):761–9.

39. Nelson R, Higgins A, Conrad J, et al. T he wide-awake approach to Dupuytren's disease: fasciectomy under local anesthetic with epinephrine. Hand (N Y) 2010;5(2):117–24.

40. Davison PG, Cobb T, Lalonde DH. The patient's perspective on carpal tunnel surgery related to the type of anesthesia: a prospective cohort study. Hand (N Y) 2013;8(1):47–53.

41. Marcus JR, Tyrone JW, Few JW, et al. Optimization of conscious sedation in plastic surgery. Plast Reconstr Surg 1999;104(5):1338–45.

42. Claxton AR, McGuire G, Chung F, et al. Evaluation of morphine versus fentanyl for postoperative analgesia after ambulatory surgical procedures. Anesth Analg 1997;84(3):509–14.

43. Zhang WY, Li Wan Po A. Analgesic efficacy of paracetamol and its combination with codeine and caffeine in surgical pain–a meta-analysis. J Clin Pharm Ther 1996;21(4):261–82.

44. Bonnefont J, Courade JP, Alloui A, et al. Antinociceptive mechanism of action of paracetamol. Drugs 2003;63(Spec No 2):1–4 [in French].

45. Mancini F, Landolfi C, Muzio M, et al. Acetaminophen down-regulates interleukin-1beta-induced nuclear factor-kappaB nuclear translocation in a human astrocytic cell line. Neurosci Lett 2003; 353(2):79–82.

46. Yancey DL, Calamia KT. Use of COX-II inhibitors for hand surgery patients. J Hand Surg Am 2008; 33(10):1909–10.

47. Yaksh TL, Malmberg AB. Spinal actions of NSAIDS in blocking spinally mediated hyperalgesia: the role of cyclooxygenase products. Agents Actions Suppl 1993;41:89–100.

48. Vane JR. Inhibition of prostaglandin synthesis as a mechanism of action for aspirin-like drugs. Nat New Biol 1971;231(25):232–5.

49. McGoldrick MD, Bailie GR. Nonnarcotic analgesics: prevalence and estimated economic impact of toxicities. Ann Pharmacother 1997;31(2):221–7.

50. Rømsing J, Møiniche S. A systematic review of COX-2 inhibitors compared with traditional NSAIDs, or different COX-2 inhibitors for post-operative pain. Acta Anaesthesiol Scand 2004;48(5):525–46.

51. Pichard CP, Laporte DM. Use of ketorolac (toradol) in hand surgery. J Hand Surg Am 2009;34(8):1549–50.

52. Kinsella J, Moffat AC, Patrick JA, et al. Ketorolac trometamol for postoperative analgesia after orthopaedic surgery. Br J Anaesth 1992;69(1):19–22.

53. Chin KR, Sundram H, Marcotte P. Bleeding risk with ketorolac after lumbar microdiscectomy. J Spinal Disord Tech 2007;20(2):123–6.

54. Richman JM, Liu SS, Courpas G, et al. Does continuous peripheral nerve block provide superior pain control to opioids? A meta-analysis. Anesth Analg 2006;102(1):248–57.

55. Rawal N, Allvin R, Amilon A, et al. Postoperative analgesia at home after ambulatory hand surgery: a controlled comparison of tramadol, metamizol, and paracetamol. Anesth Analg 2001;92(2):347–51.

56. Raffa RB. Pharmacology of oral combination analgesics: rational therapy for pain. J Clin Pharm Ther 2001;26(4):257–64.

57. Rawal N, Macquaire V, Catalá E, et al. Tramadol/paracetamol combination tablet for postoperative pain following ambulatory hand surgery: a double-blind, double-dummy, randomized, parallel-group trial. J Pain Res 2011;4:103–10.

58. Goebel S, Stehle J, Schwemmer U, et al. Interscalene brachial plexus block for open-shoulder

surgery: a randomized, double-blind, placebo-controlled trial between single-shot anesthesia and patient-controlled catheter system. Arch Orthop Trauma Surg 2010;130(4):533–40.

59. Ilfeld BM, Morey TE, Wright TW, et al. Continuous interscalene brachial plexus block for postoperative pain control at home: a randomized, double-blinded, placebo-controlled study. Anesth Analg 2003;96(4):1089–95 [table of contents].

60. Grant SA, Nielsen KC, Greengrass RA, et al. Continuous peripheral nerve block for ambulatory surgery. Reg Anesth Pain Med 2001;26(3):209–14.

61. Klein SM, Grant SA, Greengrass RA, et al. Interscalene brachial plexus block with a continuous catheter insertion system and a disposable infusion pump. Anesth Analg 2000;91(6):1473–8.

62. Ahsan ZS, Carvalho B, Yao J. Incidence of failure of continuous peripheral nerve catheters for postoperative analgesia in upper extremity surgery. J Hand Surg Am 2014;39(2):324–9.

63. Jenkins CR, Karmakar MK. An unusual complication of interscalene brachial plexus catheterization: delayed catheter migration. Br J Anaesth 2005;95(4):535–7.

64. Capdevila X, Dadure C, Bringuier S, et al. Effect of patient-controlled perineural analgesia on rehabilitation and pain after ambulatory orthopedic surgery: a multicenter randomized trial. Anesthesiology 2006;105(3):566–73.

65. Salinas FV. Location, location, location: continuous peripheral nerve blocks and stimulating catheters. Reg Anesth Pain Med 2003;28(2):79–82.

66. Wiegel M, Gottschaldt U, Hennebach R, et al. Complications and adverse effects associated with continuous peripheral nerve blocks in orthopedic patients. Anesth Analg 2007;104(6):1578–82 [table of contents].

67. Ekatodramis G, Macaire P, Borgeat A. Prolonged Horner syndrome due to neck hematoma after continuous interscalene block. Anesthesiology 2001;95(3):801–3.

68. Capdevila X, Bringuier S, Borgeat A. Infectious risk of continuous peripheral nerve blocks. Anesthesiology 2009;110(1):182–8.

69. Saraghi M, Hersh EV. Three newly approved analgesics: an update. Anesth Prog 2013;60(4):178–87.

70. Golf M, Daniels SE, Onel E. A phase 3, randomized, placebo-controlled trial of DepoFoam® bupivacaine (extended-release bupivacaine local analgesic) in bunionectomy. Adv Ther 2011;28(9):776–88.

71. Portillo J, Kamar N, Melibary S, et al. Safety of liposome extended-release bupivacaine for postoperative pain control. Front Pharmacol 2014;5:90.

72. Curley J, Castillo J, Hotz J, et al. Prolonged regional nerve blockade. Injectable biodegradable bupivacaine/polyester microspheres. Anesthesiology 1996;84(6):1401–10.

73. Masters DB, Berde CB, Dutta SK, et al. Prolonged regional nerve blockade by controlled release of local anesthetic from a biodegradable polymer matrix. Anesthesiology 1993;79(2):340–6.

74. Colombo G, Padera R, Langer R, et al. Prolonged duration local anesthesia with lipid-protein-sugar particles containing bupivacaine and dexamethasone. J Biomed Mater Res A 2005;75(2):458–64.

75. Ilfeld BM, Malhotra N, Furnish TJ, et al. Liposomal bupivacaine as a single-injection peripheral nerve block: a dose-response study. Anesth Analg 2013;117(5):1248–56.

76. Morales R, Mentz H, Newall G, et al. Use of abdominal field block injections with liposomal bupivacaine to control postoperative pain after abdominoplasty. Aesthet Surg J 2013;33(8):1148–53.

77. McAlvin JB, Padera RF, Shankarappa SA, et al. Multivesicular liposomal bupivacaine at the sciatic nerve. Biomaterials 2014;35(15):4557–64.

78. Richard BM, Newton P, Ott LR, et al. The safety of EXPAREL ® (bupivacaine liposome injectable suspension) administered by peripheral nerve block in rabbits and dogs. J Drug Deliv 2012;2012:962101.

Oncology

Preface

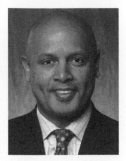

Felasfa M. Wodajo, MD
Editor

In the Oncology Section of this issue of *Orthopedic Clinics of North America*, we learn about the present and the potential future uses of PET imaging for sarcoma. Metabolic imaging, especially when combined with anatomic imaging in the form of PET/CT, has found great utility in many oncology disciplines. In "PET Imaging in Sarcoma," Drs Stephen Becher and Shervin Oskouei of Emory University explore which indications seem most promising thus far and which may turn out to be deadends. Dr Oskouei is Assistant Professor of Orthopaedic Surgery at Emory University in Atlanta, Georgia.

In "Soft Tissue Masses for the General Orthopedic Surgeon," Drs Edward Jernigan and Robert Esther of University of North Carolina (UNC) Chapel Hill survey soft tissue tumors from the perspective of the nononcologic orthopedist and point out useful findings that may help distinguish benign from malignant entities. In addition to discussing the pros and cons of the various imaging modalities available, the authors survey the basics of soft tissue sarcoma, including prognosis. Dr Esther is Associate Professor and Residency Program Director, UNC Department of Orthopaedics in Chapel Hill, North Carolina.

Felasfa M. Wodajo, MD
1625 N. George Mason, Suite 464
Arlington, VA 22205, USA

E-mail address:
wodajo@sarcoma.md

Orthop Clin N Am 46 (2015) xix
http://dx.doi.org/10.1016/j.ocl.2015.03.004
0030-5898/15/$ – see front matter © 2015 Published by Elsevier Inc.

PET Imaging in Sarcoma

Stephen Becher, MD*, Shervin Oskouei, MD

KEYWORDS

- Sarcoma • PET • PET/CT • Extremity • Soft tissue

KEY POINTS

- PET/CT scanning has evidence that it may be used in biopsy guidance, tumor detection and grading, tumor staging, therapeutic monitoring, and prognostication in sarcoma diagnosis and treatment.
- Currently the evidence does not support the routine use of PET/CT scanning in most sarcoma cases.
- Individual cases of specific histologic subtypes may benefit from PET/CT scanning for staging, biopsy guidance, and/or therapeutic monitoring.

INTRODUCTION

Extremity bone and soft tissue sarcomas are a heterogeneous group of tumors that arise from a mesenchymal origin. They are a rare group of cancers that represent less than 1% of all cancer cases. Approximately 12,000 new soft tissue and 3000 new bone sarcomas were diagnosed in America during 2014.[1] The diagnosis and treatment of extremity sarcomas has guidelines, although the heterogeneity of tumors in this group makes standardization of treatment a difficult proposition. Current guidelines call for a local MRI of the lesion and a computer tomography (CT) scan of the chest before surgery and a core needle biopsy to diagnose the histology of the tumor. Currently use of PET/CT scans is not considered as standard of care in the diagnosis and treatment of extremity sarcomas.[2,3]

PET scanning was originally performed independently from high-resolution anatomic imaging, such as CT. Before 2001 the fusion of PET and CT scanning was done with software fusion techniques and had clinical applicability limited mainly to the brain. Since 2001, however, commercially available combined CT and PET scanners have allowed the advent of combined acquisition of images and use of combined PET/CT scans is

common in areas of the body other than the brain. The standard of care is now to use combined PET/CT scan and this article assumes the use of a combined PET/CT scan.[4]

The principle of PET is that proton-rich nucleotides emit positrons via β^+ decay. In this mode a nucleus emits a positron and neutrino while reducing its atomic number by one to a more stable, less proton-rich, nucleus. The neutrino passes through matter without interacting but the positron travels only a few millimeters at most before interacting with an electron in the surrounding matter. Once the positron and electron interact they annihilate each other, giving rise to two photons of equal energy (511 keV) that travel in opposite directions. A ring of detectors around the patient allows for detection of these particular photons traveling in opposite directions with a specific energy. The detection of the dual photon events allows for indirect measurement and localization of the originating positron. The F18 isotope of fluoride is a positron emitter with a relatively long half-life, allowing it to be incorporated into the glucose analog F18-deoxyglucose. F18-deoxyglucose may be injected into a patient, taken up preferentially by abnormal oncologic tissue, and measured using a PET scanner. Doing so allows for detection of primary and metastatic malignant

The authors have nothing to disclose.
Department of Orthopedic Surgery, Emory University, 57 Executive Park South, 160-3, Atlanta, GA 30329, USA
* Corresponding author.
E-mail address: xiaobaidi@yahoo.com

Orthop Clin N Am 46 (2015) 409–415
http://dx.doi.org/10.1016/j.ocl.2015.03.001

orthopedic.theclinics.com

disease of many differing types.[5] This article evaluates the possible role of PET/CT in diagnosis and treatment of bone and soft tissue sarcomas of the extremities.

AREAS OF APPLICABILITY

PET/CT scanning has been studied in sarcoma detection and grading, biopsy guidance, sarcoma staging, therapeutic monitoring, and prognostication (**Box 1**).

Sarcoma Detection and Grading

This area is the oldest and most researched area for PET scanning in sarcoma. The standardized uptake value (SUV) is a measure of radioactivity in a specific area of interest relative to an idealized even distribution of radioactive material throughout the body. A higher SUV value means the area interrogated by the scan is more metabolically active. In general, higher-grade tumors are more metabolically active than lower grade tumors.[6] However, caution must be taken in such generalizations because high-grade tumors may have a low metabolic activity and not every highly metabolically active tumor is necessarily a malignant entity.[7]

Different studies have used different cutoffs for SUV values to determine if the SUV can predict grade. Folpe and coworkers[8] used an SUV value of greater than 7.5 as a cutoff and found 93% of tumors in this group were high-grade sarcomas, although this means that 7% of benign tumors also were in this group. At the same time 52% of all high-grade malignancies had an SUV value of less than 7.5. There was a correlation between higher SUV values in high-grade tumors and histologic findings of increased mitosis rate and cellularity.[8] Charest and coworkers[9] found that all lesions in their study of 212 bone and soft tissue sarcomas that had an SUV value of greater than 6.5 were of high grade, although many high-grade sarcomas had SUV values of less than 6.5. Meta-analysis performed by Ioannidis and Lau[7]

evaluated cutoffs of SUV greater than 2.0 and greater than 3.0 and varying levels of sensitivity and specificity for each cutoff.

Bastiaannet and coworkers[6] performed a meta-analysis of the available literature in 2004 with regards to detection of sarcomas using PET scanning. Overall sensitivity, specificity, and accuracy were found to be 91%, 85%, and 88%.[6]

Using SUV can allow for an estimation of tumor grade before biopsy (**Fig. 1**). A more metabolically active tumor is more likely to be high grade than a less metabolically active tumor, although there are enough outliers that one cannot rely on SUV values alone to determine grade. It remains a supplement to and does not replace biopsy of the lesion and histologic examination by a pathologist to determine the grade. This remains the gold standard for sarcoma grading.

Biopsy Guidance

The most interesting application of PET scanning in sarcoma is its use to direct biopsy. There are often areas of necrosis or inhomogeneity seen on MRI in a sarcoma mass. If these areas are sampled the diagnosis is subject to sampling error. This may cause the tumor to be inappropriately graded, delay diagnosis, or if there is not enough clinical suspicion, allow a sarcoma to go undiagnosed. To avoid such scenarios it has been suggested to use PET scanning as a means to determine the most metabolically active area of a tumor

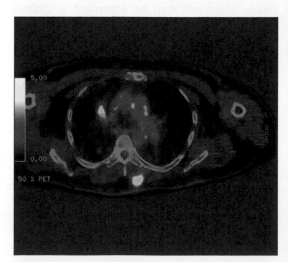

Fig. 1. PET scan of a 58-year-old man with a leiomyosarcoma in the posterior aspect of the spine. Although PET scanning can estimate the grade of a tumor with high accuracy it does not replace the need for accurate histologic diagnosis, which is the gold standard for grading any sarcoma. In addition the exact cutoffs in SUV$_{max}$ values are not standardized across studies and between institutions for which tumors are high grade.

Box 1
Areas PET/CT scanning may be useful in sarcoma diagnosis and treatment

- Sarcoma detection
- Sarcoma grading
- Sarcoma staging
- Biopsy guidance
- Therapeutic monitoring
- Prognostication

---

and direct sampling of the biopsy, whether open or percutaneous, into the area with the greatest SUV.

Park and coworkers[10] demonstrated this in a case report that demonstrated the success of this technique and showed that areas of signal inhomogeneity on MRI do not always correlate with the areas of highest SUV activity on PET scan. Hain and coworkers[11] in a case series of 20 patients had similar findings. MRI and PET scan were discordant with regards to the best region to sample 35% of the time, showing that areas of MRI inhomogeneity are not always the most metabolically active. Areas of high SUV activity had the most diagnostic yield in this series of patients.[11]

Unfortunately the evidence for such procedures remains confined to small retrospective case series and isolated case reports. The routine use of PET scans to guide biopsy cannot be advocated on this basis. However, when biopsy results are inconclusive or not consistent with the overall clinical and radiologic picture the patient may benefit from a targeted second biopsy with use of PET scan to determine the best area of a large tumor that needs to be sampled (**Fig. 2**). No

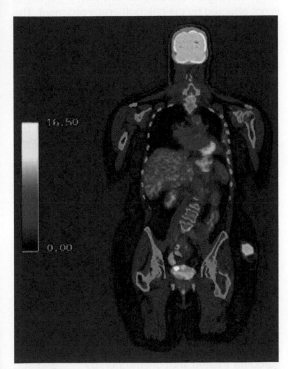

Fig. 2. PET scan in a 68-year-old woman with an undifferentiated pleomorphic sarcoma of the left buttock region. There is a highly metabolically active area superiorly and a metabolically inactive area inferiorly. The metabolically inactive area corresponded to a region of tumor that had a high degree of necrosis. Areas that are metabolically inactive may have less diagnostic yield on biopsy because of sampling error.

cost-benefit analyses exist to date in the literature for such procedures.

Sarcoma Staging

Metastasis in soft tissue and bone sarcoma is predominantly (around 75% of the time) to the lung.[12] Myxoid/round cell liposarcoma is known to have a predilection for retroperitoneal involvement and may benefit from abdominal imaging in addition to chest on initial staging.[13] Lymph node metastasis or involvement is rare, occurring in around 3% of all patients. Histologic subtypes with a predilection to lymph node involvement include synovial sarcoma, rhabdomyosarcoma, clear cell sarcoma, and epithelioid sarcoma.[14,15] Unless histology known to have nonstandard metastatic patterns is present the standard of care is for a thin-cut CT scan of the chest to evaluate for metastasis and complete staging in addition to biopsy results.[4,5]

Piperkova and coworkers[16] in a small series of 16 patients found the PET scanning revealed no new sites of metastatic disease compared with CT scan alone. Tateishi and coworkers[17] found in retrospectively evaluating 117 patients with bone or soft tissue sarcomas that overall TNM staging accuracy was 87% for combined PET/CT and conventional imaging (87%), 83% for PET/CT alone, and 77% for conventional imaging alone. The conclusion drawn was that adding PET/CT to conventional imaging can increase staging accuracy.[17]

Fuglø and coworkers[18] retrospectively reviewed 89 patients with bone and soft tissue sarcomas. The positive predictive value for lymph node metastasis was found to be only 27%. The authors concluded that PET/CT was a poor test for lymph node metastasis because of too many false-positives that would trigger unnecessary, invasive, and expensive evaluation of lymph nodes. The sensitivity, specificity, positive predictive value, and negative predictive value for distant metastasis was found to be 95%, 95%, 87%, and 98%, respectively. The authors conclude that although PET/CT was good for detection of distant metastasis, traditional CT (which has a finer CT slice than PET/CT) was better for lung metastasis.[18]

Roberge and coworkers[19] performed two studies on initial staging in soft tissue sarcomas alone. In the initial study of 75 patients there were only 1.3% of patients who were upstaged as a result of PET/CT imaging, and no patients had the management of their metastatic disease changed as a result of the PET/CT staging.[19] In the follow-up study of 109 patients, 4.5% of patients were upstaged as a result of PET/CT and 3.3% of patients had a management change as a result of the PET/CT scan. However, this had to be weighed against an equal percentage of patients who underwent a false-positive intervention with invasive procedures. In both studies the authors concluded that PET/CT scanning added little over CT scanning of the chest alone. In less than 5% of cases would management be changed and this had to be weighed against the morbidity and cost associated with false-positive results.[20]

Some theoretic advantages of PET/CT scanning in tumor staging are that it allows for imaging of the whole body rather than just an isolated CT scan and that the metabolic activity portion of the PET/CT would be able to pick up areas of potential metastasis more than CT scan alone. However, most of the evidence does not bear this out. Because the pretest probability of nonpulmonary metastasis in most sarcoma histologies is low there are often false-positive results that occur (**Fig. 3**). Also the likelihood that a positive PET/

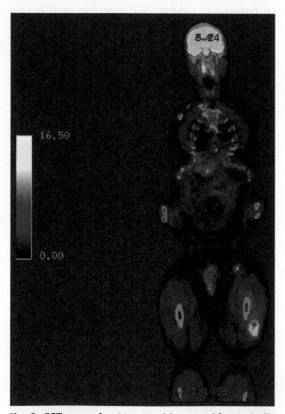

Fig. 3. PET scan of a 64-year-old man with a spindle cell neoplasm of the left thigh that also had a positive inguinal lymph node. The lymph node was biopsied in this case and was negative for metastatic disease. Because of the high number of false-positive nodes in several studies reviewed the routine use of PET scanning to determine lymph node metastasis is not recommended except in histologic subtypes with high nodal metastasis rates.

CT scan would actually change the management of a patient remains low. Given these constraints it seems clear that routine use of PET/CT scanning for staging should not be performed. Perhaps it may be useful as an adjunct in certain histologies that are more likely to have nonpulmonary metastasis, but there is little evidence for such a case currently.

Therapeutic Monitoring

Although neoadjuvant chemotherapy is a mainstay of treatment in osteosarcoma,[21] it may also be used in soft tissue sarcoma histologic subtypes that are chemosensitive.[22,23] Histologic examination of the excised specimen is correlated with increased disease-free survival and decreased local recurrence risk when tumor necrosis exceeds 95% in osteosarcoma.[24] One study found a similar finding in soft tissue sarcoma.[25] Although this has not been reproduced consistently, PET scanning has been investigated as a tool to monitor chemotherapy response in soft tissue and bony sarcomas, ideally allowing the clinician early warning before surgical excision if the tumor is not affected by the chemotherapy regiment. The theoretic advantage would allow chemotherapy regiments either to be changed or discontinued with earlier surgery if there is a nonresponse, although no study to date has shown this. In addition, the response or lack thereof would be useful in counseling patients on their overall prognosis.

In monitoring treatment response there are three major variables measured on the PET scans. The first is SUV_{max}, which is the maximal value of the SUV uptake. The second is metabolic tumor volume (MTV; also called gross tumor volume), which is the size of the tumor that is metabolically active, often taken as a percent of SUV_{max}.[26] The third is the total lesion glycolysis, which is the average SUV of the tumor multiplied by the MTV.[27] All three indices are measuring the overall metabolic activity of the tumor, which is then compared between scans done before chemotherapy and at some time point after treatment with chemotherapy.

Multiple studies have evaluated the effectiveness of PET scanning in monitoring therapeutic response. PET scanning has been found to be effective at predicting histologic necrosis in osteosarcoma treated with chemotherapy[28–30] and soft tissue sarcoma treated with chemotherapy.[30–32] PET scanning is also effective at predicting survival after chemotherapy in soft tissue sarcoma.[33] What the studies do not show with any convincing certainty is the appropriate time point at which to measure the markers: after one cycle, after two cycles, or at the end of treatment. Certainly

---

Box 2
Pros and cons for PET/CT

Pros	Cons
Allows biopsy guidance to active metabolic areas	Clinical suspicion of aggressive-appearing lesions directs physicians to resample equivocal biopsy results
Allows evaluation of chemotherapy response before resection and histologic examination	Cutoffs for stopping chemotherapy by PET/CT are poorly defined
Allows for evaluation of lymph nodes and nonpulmonary sites of metastatic disease	PET/CT has false-positives that cause unnecessary biopsies and procedures to be performed
Allows for noninvasive grading of tumors	PET/CT does not obviate biopsy, which is the gold standard for tumor grading

---

measuring at the end of treatment provides little information because the histologic examination after surgical excision provides the gold standard for prognosis. The cutoffs for various markers are poorly defined and vary from study to study. The greater the decrease in glucose activity portends a better prognosis, although the clinician must weigh how much information will be gleaned mid-therapy.

Prognostication

The ability for PET/CT to predict outcome before any chemotherapy has also been investigated. PET/CT has been shown to predict progression-free survival in soft tissue sarcomas[34] and overall survival and local control in soft tissue sarcomas.[35] PET/CT has been shown, likewise, to predict metastasis-free survival in osteosarcoma.[36] There remains, as with the studies for treatment monitoring, a lack of standardization with regards to the indices measured and cutoff values between studies.

PET/CT scanning does have the ability to prognosticate before beginning chemotherapy, although there are no studies comparing PET/CT prognostic ability with general staging done with local imaging, CT chest, and biopsy results. It is the authors' opinion that the current prognostic information from PET/CT scan would not supersede or add additional information to that gained from a normal staging work-up. High-grade lesions on biopsy have high SUV_{max}, MTV, or total lesion glycolysis. The biopsy needs to be done no matter the PET/CT result and so makes the prognostic ability of PET/CT redundant in the authors' opinion.

AN OUNCE OF COMMON SENSE

There were no cost-effectiveness studies in any of the five categories where PET/CT scanning may be used in sarcoma diagnosis and treatment. The overall impression from the studies performed is that although there are things PET/CT scan can do, perhaps there is little additional value added in doing them (**Box 2**). Tumor grade is best determined by histologic examination and thus PET/CT is redundant if used to help predict grade. Staging is best done with conventional CT scan for most histologic types, given the high rate of false-positives on several studies. Certain histologic subtypes that have a propensity for nonpulmonary metastasis may benefit from PET/CT scanning in addition to traditional CT of the chest to give a higher pretest probability and prevent false-positive results. Therapeutic monitoring may have some value in allowing clinicians to determine when to abort chemotherapy in a nonresponder. Values measured by the PET/CT scan must be researched and standardized, however, before the technology is used to abort chemotherapy early. In addition, the cost of multiple PET/CT scans needs to be weighed in a prospective manner before any change to standard of care.

Currently PET/CT scans should not be used routinely in the diagnosis and treatment of sarcomas. As further studies are done, this may change, but the marginal benefit that the studies may provide does not currently outweigh the cost to the patient in possible unnecessary invasive procedures and in the cost of the test itself.

REFERENCES

1. American Cancer Society. Cancer facts and figures 2014. Atlanta (GA): American Cancer Society; 2014.
2. Grimer R, Judson I, Peake D, et al. Guidelines for the management of soft tissue sarcomas. Sarcoma 2010;2010:506182.
3. Casali PG, Jost L, Sleijfer S, et al. Soft tissue sarcomas: ESMO clinical recommendations for diagnosis, treatment and follow-up. Ann Oncol 2009; 20(Suppl 4):132–6.

4. Townsend DW. Positron emission tomography/computed tomography. Semin Nucl Med 2008;38(3):152–66.

5. Blokland JA, Trindev P, Stokkel MP, et al. Positron emission tomography: a technical introduction for clinicians. Eur J Radiol 2002;44(1):70–5.

6. Bastiaannet E, Groen H, Jager PL, et al. The value of FDG-PET in the detection, grading and response to therapy of soft tissue and bone sarcomas; a systematic review and meta-analysis. Cancer Treat Rev 2004;30(1):83–101.

7. Ioannidis JP, Lau J. 18F-FDG PET for the diagnosis and grading of soft-tissue sarcoma: a meta-analysis. J Nucl Med 2003;44(5):717–24.

8. Folpe AL, Lyles RH, Sprouse JT, et al. (F-18) fluorodeoxyglucose positron emission tomography as a predictor of pathologic grade and other prognostic variables in bone and soft tissue sarcoma. Clin Cancer Res 2000;6(4):1279–87.

9. Charest M, Hickeson M, Lisbona R, et al. FDG PET/CT imaging in primary osseous and soft tissue sarcomas: a retrospective review of 212 cases. Eur J Nucl Med Mol Imaging 2009;36(12):1944–51.

10. Park JH, Park EK, Kang CH, et al. Intense accumulation of 18F-FDG, not enhancement on MRI, helps to guide the surgical biopsy accurately in soft tissue tumors. Ann Nucl Med 2009;23(10):887–9.

11. Hain SF, O'Doherty MJ, Bingham J, et al. Can FDG PET be used to successfully direct preoperative biopsy of soft tissue tumours? Nucl Med Commun 2003;24(11):1139–43.

12. Billingsley KG, Lewis JJ, Leung DH, et al. Multifactorial analysis of the survival of patients with distant metastasis arising from primary extremity sarcoma. Cancer 1999;85(2):389–95.

13. Moreau LC, Turcotte R, Ferguson P, et al. Myxoid \ round cell liposarcoma (MRCLS) revisited: an analysis of 418 primarily managed cases. Ann Surg Oncol 2012;19(4):1081–8.

14. Fong Y, Coit DG, Woodruff JM, et al. Lymph node metastasis from soft tissue sarcoma in adults. Analysis of data from a prospective database of 1772 sarcoma patients. Ann Surg 1993;217(1):72–7.

15. Riad S, Griffin AM, Liberman B, et al. Lymph node metastasis in soft tissue sarcoma in an extremity. Clin Orthop Relat Res 2004;(426):129–34.

16. Piperkova E, Mikhaeil M, Mousavi A, et al. Impact of PET and CT in PET/CT studies for staging and evaluating treatment response in bone and soft tissue sarcomas. Clin Nucl Med 2009;34(3):146–50.

17. Tateishi U, Yamaguchi U, Seki K, et al. Bone and soft-tissue sarcoma: preoperative staging with fluorine 18 fluorodeoxyglucose PET/CT and conventional imaging. Radiology 2007;245(3):839–47.

18. Fuglø HM, Jørgensen SM, Loft A, et al. The diagnostic and prognostic value of ^{18}F-FDG PET/CT in the initial assessment of high-grade bone and soft tissue sarcoma. A retrospective study of 89 patients. Eur J Nucl Med Mol Imaging 2012;39(9):1416–24.

19. Roberge D, Hickeson M, Charest M, et al. Initial McGill experience with fluorodeoxyglucose pet/ct staging of soft-tissue sarcoma. Curr Oncol 2010;17(6):18–22.

20. Roberge D, Vakilian S, Alabed YZ, et al. FDG PET/CT in initial staging of adult soft-tissue sarcoma. Sarcoma 2012;2012:960194.

21. Bielack S, Carrle D, Jost L, et al. Osteosarcoma: ESMO clinical recommendations for diagnosis, treatment and follow-up. Ann Oncol 2008;19(Suppl 2):ii94–6.

22. Sleijfer S, Ouali M, van Glabbeke M, et al. Prognostic and predictive factors for outcome to first-line ifosfamide-containing chemotherapy for adult patients with advanced soft tissue sarcomas: an exploratory, retrospective analysis on large series from the European Organization for Research and Treatment of Cancer-Soft Tissue and Bone Sarcoma Group (EORTC-STBSG). Eur J Cancer 2010;46(1):72–83.

23. Jones RL, Fisher C, Al-Muderis O, et al. Differential sensitivity of liposarcoma subtypes to chemotherapy. Eur J Cancer 2005;41(18):2853–60.

24. Bramer JA, van Linge JH, Grimer RJ, et al. Prognostic factors in localized extremity osteosarcoma: a systematic review. Eur J Surg Oncol 2009;35(10):1030–6.

25. Eilber FC, Rosen G, Eckardt J, et al. Treatment-induced pathologic necrosis: a predictor of local recurrence and survival in patients receiving neoadjuvant therapy for high-grade extremity soft tissue sarcomas. J Clin Oncol 2001;19:3203.

26. Biehl KJ, Kong FM, Dehdashti F, et al. 18F-FDG PET definition of gross tumor volume for radiotherapy of non-small cell lung cancer: is a single standardized uptake value threshold approach appropriate? J Nucl Med 2006;47:1808–12.

27. Larson SM, Erdi Y, Akhurst T, et al. Tumor treatment response based on visual and quantitative changes in global tumor glycolysis using PET-FDG imaging. The visual response score and the change in total lesion glycolysis. Clin Positron Imaging 1999;2:159–71.

28. Im HJ, Kim TS, Park SY, et al. Prediction of tumour necrosis fractions using metabolic and volumetric 18F-FDG PET/CT indices, after one course and at the completion of neoadjuvant chemotherapy, in children and young adults with osteosarcoma. Eur J Nucl Med Mol Imaging 2012;39(1):39–49.

29. Hongtao L, Hui Z, Bingshun W, et al. 18F-FDG positron emission tomography for the assessment of histological response to neoadjuvant chemotherapy in osteosarcomas: a meta-analysis. Surg Oncol 2012;21(4):e165–70.

30. Eary JF, Conrad EU, O'Sullivan J, et al. Sarcoma midtherapy [F-18]fluorodeoxyglucose positron emission

tomography (FDG PET) and patient outcome. J Bone Joint Surg Am 2014;96(2):152–8.

31. Benz MR, Czernin J, Allen-Auerbach MS, et al. FDG-PET/CT imaging predicts histopathologic treatment responses after the initial cycle of neoadjuvant chemotherapy in high-grade soft-tissue sarcomas. Clin Cancer Res 2009;15(8):2856–63.

32. Evilevitch V, Weber WA, Tap WD, et al. Reduction of glucose metabolic activity is more accurate than change in size at predicting histopathologic response to neoadjuvant therapy in high-grade soft-tissue sarcomas. Clin Cancer Res 2008;14(3):715–20.

33. Herrmann K, Benz MR, Czernin J, et al. 18F-FDG-PET/CT Imaging as an early survival predictor in patients with primary high-grade soft tissue sarcomas undergoing neoadjuvant therapy. Clin Cancer Res 2012;18(7):2024–31.

34. Choi ES, Ha SG, Kim HS, et al. Total lesion glycolysis by 18F-FDG PET/CT is a reliable predictor of prognosis in soft-tissue sarcoma. Eur J Nucl Med Mol Imaging 2013;40(12):1836–42.

35. Schwarzbach MH, Hinz U, Dimitrakopoulou-Strauss A, et al. Prognostic significance of preoperative [18-F] fluorodeoxyglucose (FDG) positron emission tomography (PET) imaging in patients with resectable soft tissue sarcomas. Ann Surg 2005;241(2):286–94.

36. Byun BH, Kong CB, Park J, et al. Initial metabolic tumor volume measured by 18F-FDG PET/CT can predict the outcome of osteosarcoma of the extremities. J Nucl Med 2013;54(10):1725–32.

Soft Tissue Masses for the General Orthopedic Surgeon

Edward W. Jernigan, MD[a], Robert J. Esther, MD, MSc[b],*

KEYWORDS

- Soft tissue sarcoma of extremities • Tumor • Soft tissue mass • Unplanned resection

KEY POINTS

- Soft tissue sarcoma should be on the differential diagnosis for any patient presenting with a soft tissue mass.
- Soft tissue sarcomas do not always display aggressive clinical behavior. Although the classic description is an enlarging, subfascial mass greater than 5 cm, some sarcomas are superficial and have a very indolent growth rate.
- Patients with suspected soft tissue sarcomas should be referred to a specialty center with a multidisciplinary sarcoma team before biopsy is performed. Although less invasive than open biopsies, even percutaneous biopsies can complicate potential resections. Furthermore, some biopsies performed before referral are unnecessary, and can lead to unnecessary patient anxiety.
- Patients who undergo unplanned resection of a soft tissue sarcoma should be referred to a specialty center for consideration of reexcision and radiation therapy.
- Delays in diagnosis and unplanned resections have been associated with worse patient outcomes.

INTRODUCTION

Soft tissue masses are commonly encountered in general orthopedic clinics. Differentiation between benign and malignant soft tissue masses is challenging. When a systematic approach is applied to the workup for soft tissue masses, however, the chances of a delay in diagnosis or an unplanned resection are minimized. Early referral to a tumor center with an experienced multidisciplinary team for further workup of masses suspicious for soft tissue sarcoma leads to better patient outcomes.[1,2]

There are approximately 11,000 new cases of soft tissue sarcoma diagnosed each year, which account for approximately 1% of all cancers diagnosed in the United States.[3] Soft tissue sarcomas represent a heterogeneous group of malignancies. The many subtypes of soft tissue sarcomas share a common mesenchymal tissue of origin. Despite this similarity, soft tissue sarcomas exhibit a wide range of histologic findings and clinical behavior. This heterogeneity leads to diagnostic and therapeutic challenges.[4] Soft tissue sarcomas develop in patients of all ages with a slight male predominance.[3] These tumors are most likely to occur in the lower extremity, followed by the upper extremities and trunk.[5]

CLINICAL PRESENTATION AND EVALUATION

The clinical presentation of a soft tissue sarcoma is nonspecific and similar to that of many benign

Disclosures: None (E.W. Jernigan); Musculoskeletal Transplant Foundation (member of Medical Board of Trustees) (R.J. Esther).
[a] Department of Orthopaedics, UNC School of Medicine, University of North Carolina, 3147 Bioinformatics Building, 130 Mason Farm Road, Chapel Hill, NC 27599-7055, USA; [b] Department of Orthopaedics, University of North Carolina, Campus Box 7055, 3155 Bioinformatics Building, Chapel Hill, NC 27599, USA
* Corresponding author.
E-mail address: bob@med.unc.edu

orthopedic.theclinics.com

masses. Despite the frequently aggressive histo-logic nature and propensity for metastasis of this heterogeneous class of tumors, soft tissue sar-comas are often painless. When evaluating a pa-tient with a soft tissue mass, a thorough history should be obtained that specifically notes the chronicity of the mass, changes in size or appear-ance, and the nature of the discovery of the mass. Constitutional symptoms are uncommon in pa-tients with soft tissue sarcomas and thus a patient who appears healthy may indeed be harboring a soft tissue sarcoma.[4,6] Several common diagno-ses and their salient clinical features are described in **Table 1**. The key to avoiding unplanned resec-tions and misdiagnoses is for the clinician to as-sume that all soft tissues are potentially malignant.

A detailed medical history should be attained, taking specific note of any history of prior masses or cancer. Lymphoma, multiple myeloma, and car-cinomas (most commonly lung and renal) can all manifest as soft tissue masses. A history of radia-tion therapy is a known risk factor for developing a soft tissue sarcoma.[7] The patient should be screened for a personal or family history of genetic conditions associated with increased risk of devel-oping soft tissue sarcomas. Li-Fraumeni syn-drome is a germline mutation in tumor protein 53 that predisposes a patient to developing multiple cancers at a young age.[8] Increased rates of soft tissue sarcomas are seen in patients with Gardner syndrome, also known as familial polyposis coli. Neurofibromatosis type I is a defect in the tumor suppressor gene NF1 on chromosome 17 that is inherited in an autosomal dominant fashion. Patients with neurofibromatosis can develop malignant peripheral nerve sheath tumors. An enlarging, increasingly painful neurofibroma should raise the suspicion of this development.

A thorough physical examination is a key part of the workup for a soft tissue mass. The patient should have the implicated extremity fully exposed, as well as the contralateral extremity to allow for the detection of subtle asymmetries. The size and depth of the mass should be noted. Larger than 5 cm is a risk factor for malignancy. Masses that are adherent to the fascia, or are located deep to the fascia, have an increased like-lihood of being malignant. A mass that is mobile with the nearby musculature relaxed, and remains mobile when the musculature contracted is likely to be superficial in nature.[9] A neurovascular exam-ination should be performed and compared with the contralateral side. A positive Tinel sign at the mass is suggestive of a peripheral nerve sheath tumor.

The skin around the mass should be closely inspected. A mass with cutaneous ulceration is more likely to be a skin cancer, such as a squa-mous cell carcinoma, than a sarcoma. However, this finding can be seen in soft tissue sarcomas that have become large enough to be fungating. The presence of axillary or groin freckling, as well as café au lait spots, may be present in patients with neurofibromatosis. Tenderness, erythema, and fluctuance are characteristic of an abscess. A palpable or audible thrill indicates a vascular lesion, such as an aneurysm. In the setting of trauma or a coagulopathic state, a hematoma can manifest as a soft tissue mass. In these sce-narios, the presence of ecchymosis should be assessed on examination. In the absence of ecchymosis, a diagnosis of hematoma should not be made without further work-up. Care should be taken to assess for lymphadenopathy. Promi-nent lymphadenopathy is a possible finding in lym-phoma; some soft tissue sarcomas, however, do have the capacity to metastasize via the lymphatic system.

RADIOGRAPHIC FINDINGS

Although plain radiographs are a part of the work up for most soft tissue masses, findings are most often nonspecific. However, there are several find-ings that are characteristic of some soft tissue masses. Phleboliths are smooth, round, radio-dense calcifications within venous structures that are suggestive of hemangiomas, the most com-mon soft tissue tumor in children (**Fig. 3**). Lipomas, the most common soft tissue tumor in adults, may demonstrate an area of increased radiolucency within a more radiodense area of skeletal muscle when they are intramuscular (**Fig. 4**). Mature-appearing trabecular bone around the periphery of a soft tissue mass in the setting of recent trauma to the area is suggestive of myositis ossificans (**Fig. 5**). In this clinical setting, a CT scan would be an appropriate next step to demonstrate pe-ripheral ossification of the lesion. Occasionally, soft tissue sarcomas can demonstrate central, disorganized patterns of mineralization on radio-graph (**Fig. 6**). It is uncommon for soft tissue sar-comas to cause changes to adjacent bone. However, when they do, it may take the form of cortical thickening, periosteal reaction, or bony erosion.[10]

Ultrasound can be a helpful tool for character-ization of superficial soft tissue masses, particu-larly in differentiating cystic versus solid lesions. Ultrasound can also be used to monitor a soft tis-sue mass through time to assess for change in size. Advantages of ultrasound compared with cross-sectional modalities include the lack of radi-ation exposure, decreased time to complete the study, and cost. Disadvantages of ultrasound include the operator-dependent nature of ultrasound examinations, which may complicate the reproducibility of size measurements. Additionally, in patients ultimately diagnosed with a soft tissue tumors, ultrasound has been shown to yield an incorrect initial diagnosis nearly one-quarter of the time, with an erroneous diagnosis of hematoma being the most common error. The finding of a noncystic, nonlipomatous lesion on ultrasound should prompt further evaluation.[11]

MRI is a powerful tool in the assessment of soft tissue masses. It provides excellent spatial resolution and tissue types can often be differentiated by their signal characteristics. The administration of gadolinium allows for differentiation between cystic and solid lesions. In conjunction with the history, physical examination, and other radiographic studies, MRI allows for diagnosis of many soft tissue masses without a biopsy. Lesions that may be diagnosed without tissue sampling are said to be determinate lesions and include, but are not limited to, lipomas, hemangiomas, ganglion and synovial cysts, myositis ossificans, and pigmented villonodular synovitis.[12] **Table 1** contains brief descriptions of key radiographic features of several common benign soft tissue masses. Soft tissue sarcomas enhance with the administration of contrast and usually respect fascial boundaries. It is rare for soft tissue sarcomas to be intraarticular. Lesions hypointense relative to muscle on T1 sequences and hyperintense on T2 sequences are concerning but not specific for soft tissue sarcomas (**Fig. 7**).[12]

On completion of radiographic studies, the diagnostician assesses the available data. If a confident diagnosis cannot be established based on the available clinical and radiographic data, the lesion is considered indeterminate and arrangements should be made for tissue sampling at a center with a multidisciplinary sarcoma team (**Fig. 8**). The diagnosis of hematoma should be made judiciously. Cases of soft tissue sarcomas masquerading as hematomas are well described and associated with delays in treatment and adverse outcomes (**Fig. 9**).[6,13] Traumatic hemorrhage generally tracks along fascial planes, leading to subcutaneous ecchymosis. In contrast, soft tissue sarcomas may be characterized by intratumoral hemorrhage, which is generally contained within a tumor pseudocapsule. The difficulty in differentiating hematomas from soft tissue sarcomas underscores the importance of obtaining appropriate imaging because MRIs without contrast do not allow for differentiation of these diagnoses. Clinicians should have a low threshold to refer for tissue sampling when differentiating between hematomas and soft tissue sarcomas, particularly in the absence of a history of trauma or ecchymosis on examination.

BIOPSY

In contrast to malignant bone tumors that have suggestive radiographic features, soft tissue sarcomas often present (clinically and radiographically) in a nonspecific manner. This underscores the importance of a thoughtfully planned biopsy to establish a diagnosis. Tissue sampling may be performed in a percutaneous or open manner. Regardless of the technique chosen for biopsy, consideration should be provided for the surgical approach that would be indicated for any limb-sparring procedure in the event of a diagnosis of a soft tissue sarcoma. In percutaneous biopsies, malignant cells may contaminate the biopsy tract and these tracts are often resected during the definitive surgery.[14] To prevent contamination of adjacent compartments or neurovascular bundles, which can lead to increased morbidity for the patient, communication between the treating surgeon and the musculoskeletal radiologist is essential. Similarly, open biopsies, which have the potential contaminate any exposed tissue in the approach, should be performed only by the surgeon who will provide definitive treatment.[15]

Advantages of performing a percutaneous biopsy, such as a fine-needle aspiration (FNA) or core needle biopsy (CNB), in lieu of an open biopsy include decreased costs, decreased patient morbidity, less subcutaneous hematoma formation, and the avoidance of a surgical procedure. During the past several decades, FNA has been largely replaced by CNB due to the increased sensitivity and specificity associated with CNB relative to FNA. This is related to the preservation of tissue architecture and increased amount of tissue delivered from CNB.[16,17] CNB has been shown in multiple studies to have sensitivities and specificities of greater than 90%.[18,19] Image guidance yields more accurate results than does non–image-guided CNB.[20]

Open biopsy remains the most sensitive and specific technique for diagnosis of suspected soft tissue sarcomas. It is used in cases of inadequate sampling after percutaneous techniques, or when there is discordance between pathologic specimens and clinical presentation or imaging studies. Open biopsy has been consistently shown to be more accurate than percutaneous techniques.[17,21] Open biopsies allow for direct visualization of the mass, and intraoperative frozen section sampling helps ensure an adequate specimen has been collected. When planning an open

Table 1
Clinical and radiographic features of selected common soft tissue masses

Diagnosis	History	Physical Examination	Radiograph	MRI[12]	Other Notes
Abscess	Painful, rapid onset History of prior abscess +/– fever	Erythema, warmth, tenderness, fluctuance	Nonspecific mass effect	Rim enhancement with administration of contrast May be loculated	Elevated inflammatory markers
Aneurysm	History of trauma common May be congenital More common in elderly patients	Compressible, pulsatile Popliteal fossa common site	+/– calcification of portions of vessel wall	Vessel enlarged in area of clinical concern Given vascular nature of this lesion, it enhances with contrast	Pseudoaneurysms more common than true aneurysms
Ganglion cyst	Mass may fluctuate in size Wrist common location	Mobile, tense but compressible May arise from capsules, tendon sheaths Transilluminates	Nonspecific mass effect	Rim-enhancing homogeneous lesion with intralesional signal intensity similar to that of water (dark on T1, bright on T2)	Classic presentation is dorsal wrist ganglion
Hemangioma	Dependent or activity-related fluctuations in size Female predominance	Soft, compressible Vascular ectasia may be present	Phleboliths (see **Fig. 3**)	Enhancing heterogeneous mass with characteristic serpentine appearance related to multiple vessels	Most common soft tissue mass in children
Hematoma	History of trauma Bleeding diathesis	Ecchymosis, warmth	Nonspecific mass effect	Nonenhancing heterogeneous mass Areas of high T1 signal represent ongoing hemorrhage	Soft tissue sarcomas may be erroneously diagnosed as hematomas on ultrasound and MRI (see **Fig. 9**)

Lipoma	Usually painless mass without rapid changes in size May cause symptoms from compression of neurovascular structures	Soft, mobile, nontender	Area of increased radiolucency within a more radiodense area of skeletal muscle (see **Fig. 4**)	Isointense with fat on all sequences (**Fig. 1**) Presence of fibrous degeneration, broad septations, or nodularity merit further evaluation with tissue sampling (**Fig. 2**)	Most common superficial mass in adults
Myositis ossificans	History of trauma Most common age in 20s Initially painful	Tenderness early in the course Quads and brachialis most common sites	Well-defined calcification around periphery of mass (see **Fig. 5**)	Decreased signal around periphery of lesion consistent with peripheral calcification pattern	CT more helpful for evaluating peripheral calcification of lesion
Neurofibroma	Most common in patients with neurofibromatosis +/- pain	Firm, +/- tenderness Positive Tinel sign at the mass Mobility in the transverse plane but not in the longitudinal plane	Nonspecific mass effect	Enhancing heterogeneous lesion Target sign on T2 sequencing described as circumferential area of high signal (myxoid tissue) around a center of low signal (nerve fibers)	Serial MRI may be used to monitor for degeneration to malignancy
Synovial cyst (Baker cyst)	Mass located in popliteal fossa +/- pain Fluctuates in size Associated with intraarticular pathology	Popliteal fossa Tense, compressible Clinically similar to ganglion	Nonspecific mass effect +/- Calcifications	Nonenhancing homogeneous lesion with signal intensity similar to that of water (dark on T1, bright on T2)	Communicates with joint Rupture of Baker cyst can lead to local pain

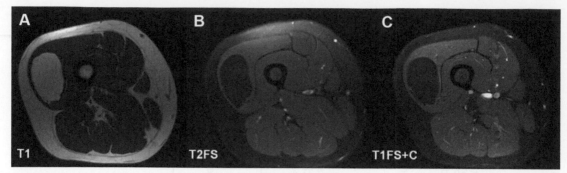

Fig. 1. Intramuscular lipoma. MRI: T1 (*A*), T2FS (*B*), T1FS+C (*C*). Note the mass is isointense to subcutaneous fat on all sequences and the lack of contrast enhancement.

biopsy, transverse incisions should be avoided. Meticulous hemostasis must be maintained to avoid formation of a hematoma that may track along subcutaneous tissue or intermuscular planes, thereby contaminating adjacent tissue with malignant cells. Dissection should be minimized by taking a direct approach to the tumor. Neurovascular bundles and adjacent compartments should not be exposed unless absolutely necessary. In high-risk areas where contamination may eliminate patients from consideration of a limb salvage procedure, such as the axilla, popliteal fossa, or carpal tunnel, open biopsies should be avoided. Arthroscopy may lead to contamination of an entire joint and is, therefore, not an appropriate method for biopsy of an intraarticular soft tissue mass.[22]

Failure to carefully plan the approach for any type of biopsy may complicate definitive treatment, possibly eliminating patients from consideration of a limb salvage procedure.

UNPLANNED RESECTIONS

Highlighting the importance of a methodical approach to the workup for a soft tissue mass

are clinical data suggesting that unplanned resections of soft tissue sarcomas complicate treatment and are associated with adverse patient outcomes. Excisional biopsies of indeterminate lesions before referral to a sarcoma specialty center should be avoided (see **Fig. 7**). Up to one-half of all patients who undergo unplanned total excision of a soft tissue sarcoma will have residual tumor in the surgical bed.[23,24] Local recurrence and survival rates after reexcision following unplanned excision of small, superficial sarcomas have been shown to be no worse than planned excision.[25] However, local recurrence rates are 2 to 3 times higher in patients who undergo unplanned excision of high-grade tumors.[24,26] Patients who undergo unplanned excision of high-grade sarcomas are more likely to develop metastatic disease and have been shown to have higher mortality rates relative to patients who undergo planned excision.[24,27]

Patients who undergo unplanned excision of a soft tissue sarcoma should be referred to a tumor center with an experienced multidisciplinary team for consideration of reexcision and radiation therapy. Reexcision of the surgical bed has been shown to lead to improved local control rates.[28]

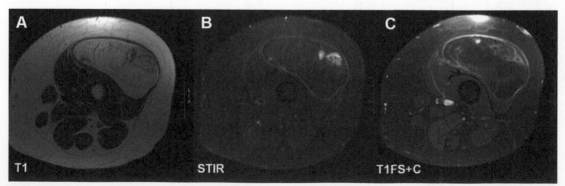

Fig. 2. Atypical lipomatous tumor. MRI: T1 (*A*), STIR (*B*), T1FS+C (*C*). Note the stranding and contrast enhancement of the mass.

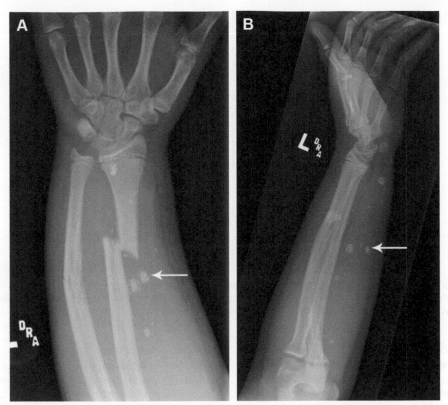

Fig. 3. Phleboliths within a hemangioma. Anteroposterior (*A*) and lateral (*B*) radiographs demonstrating phleboliths (*arrows*) seen in a pediatric patient with a forearm hemangioma in the setting of a both-bone forearm fracture.

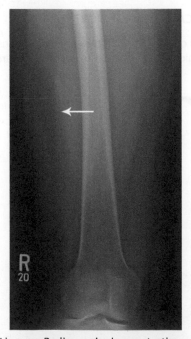

Fig. 4. Lipoma. Radiograph demonstrating a lateral thigh lipoma. Note the region of radiolucency (*arrow*) passing over it within skeletal muscle.

Five-year survival rates of over 90% have been demonstrated at centers with an aggressive protocol of reexcision. Histologic high-grade, lesions deep to the fascia and presence of metastasis are poor prognostic indicators and are associated with increased 5-year mortality rates after reexcision.[29]

PROGNOSIS

Prognosis of soft tissue sarcomas is primarily characterized by local recurrence rate, distant metastasis, and mortality. At 5 years, primary soft tissue sarcomas of the extremities have a local recurrence rate of 6% to 17%, metastatic disease rate of 22% to 36%, and mortality rate of 24% to 33%.[30–33] Operative margin has been demonstrated to be the most important treatment factor and achieving negative margins is associated with decreased rates of local recurrence.[31,34] Histologic high-grade tumors are associated with increased local recurrence, metastasis, and mortality.[29,31,35] Soft tissue sarcomas that are deep to the fascia and larger than 5 cm carry a worse prognosis.[29,31] Malignant tumor ulceration is a

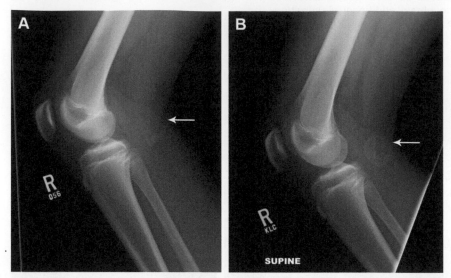

Fig. 5. Progressive heterotopic ossification in a 14-year-old boy. (*A*) Radiograph taken at patient's initial clinic visit. (*B*) Radiograph taken 3 months later. Note the interval increase in mineralization of the mass and the characteristic circumferential ossification with a lucent center (*arrows*).

poor prognostic indicator. These patients have worse survival rates and higher incidences of metastasis at the time of presentation.[36] Radiation-induced soft tissue sarcoma is associated with a higher risk of local recurrence and metastasis.[7] Bony invasion is uncommon and associated with increased mortality.[10] Older patients are at higher risk for recurrence of disease.[37]

The most common site for metastatic disease that arises via hematogenous spread of soft tissue sarcomas is the lungs. Several soft tissue sarcoma subtypes have shown a predilection to metastasize via the lymphatic system, including rhabdomyosarcoma, angiosarcoma, clear-cell sarcoma, epithelioid sarcoma, and synovial sarcoma. There is consideration for sentinel node biopsy when any of these diagnoses are established. Myxoid liposarcomas may metastasize to nonpulmonary sites, such as the abdomen, and may benefit from routine surveillance with CT scans of the abdomen.[4]

SURGICAL MANAGEMENT

Several oncologic principles should be considered for surgical management of soft tissue sarcomas.

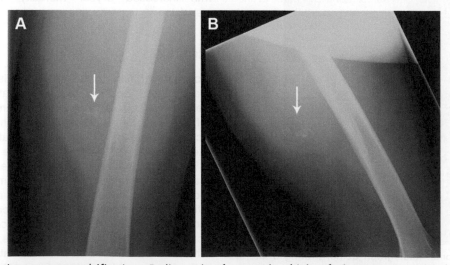

Fig. 6. Soft tissue sarcoma calcifications. Radiographs of a posterior thigh soft tissue sarcoma (alveolar soft part sarcoma) demonstrating irregular calcifications (*arrows*).

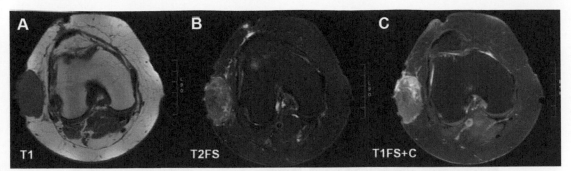

Fig. 7. Superficial soft tissue sarcoma with nonspecific radiologic findings: T1 (*A*), T2FS (*B*), T1FS+C (*C*). MRI from a 65-year-old woman who presented with a superficial soft tissue mass. This patient underwent unplanned resection (excisional biopsy) before referral to a sarcoma specialty center, which complicates treatment of soft tissue sarcomas.

It is worth repeating that any open biopsy of a soft tissue mass should be performed by the surgeon who will provide definitive surgical treatment in the event of a malignant diagnosis. As noted previously, incisions should be longitudinal and transverse incisions should be avoided. If a tourniquet is used, compressive bandages should be avoided, and gravity exsanguination should be used in these cases. Meticulous hemostasis should be maintained throughout the procedure given the possibility of contamination of hematomas with malignant cells. If it is decided to leave a drain, it should exit in line with the excision because this allows for the tract to be incorporated into future excisions if necessary.[22] Historically, percutaneous biopsy tracts have been excised during the definitive procedure. However, recent evidence comparing patients who did not undergo excision of the biopsy tract demonstrated no difference in local recurrence relative to historical controls.[38]

As originally described by Enneking, surgical resection of soft tissue masses is classified as intralesional, marginal, wide, and radical (**Table 2**). In an effort to balance the often competing interests of providing an appropriate oncologic resection and preservation of function of the limb, most primary soft tissue sarcomas are widely

excised. Amputations are generally reserved for cases in which obtaining negative margins will not allow for salvage of the vital neurovascular structures of the limb or when function will be superior with an amputation. In the past several decades, the rate of amputation for treatment of primary soft tissue sarcomas of the extremities has been decreasing.[5] Multiple studies have shown no difference in survival rates between limb salvage techniques verses amputation.[33,39] Epineural dissection has been demonstrated to be a safe technique that facilitates limb salvage, in particular in cases in which the soft tissue sarcoma abuts the sciatic nerve.[40] Some centers advocate for plastic surgery involvement for closure, particularly in the setting of irradiated tissue, with one study noting a trend toward decreased reoperation rates.[41]

RADIATION THERAPY

All patients diagnosed with soft tissue sarcomas should be considered for radiation therapy in a multidisciplinary setting. Radiation therapy has been shown to decrease local recurrence rates in adult and pediatric patients.[42,43] There is no difference in the rate of local recurrence with preoperative verses postoperative radiation. Preoperative

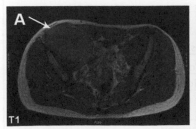
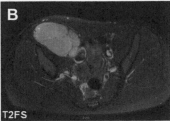
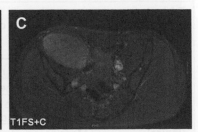

Fig. 8. MRI of soft tissue mass with nonspecific signal characteristics (*arrow*): T1 (*A*), T2FS (*B*), T1FS+C (*C*). Given the indeterminate nature of the mass, this patient underwent biopsy that demonstrated a schwannoma.

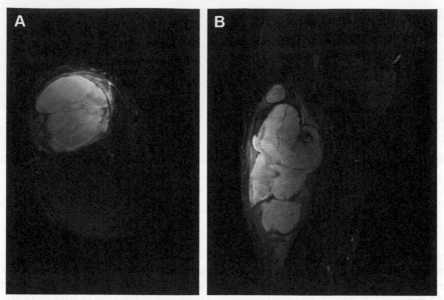

Fig. 9. High-grade pleomorphic sarcoma initially diagnosed and treated as hematoma, MRI axial (*A*) and sagittal (*B*) images (T2FS). MRI without contrast performed at a referring facility, limiting the diagnostic utility of the study.

radiation therapy is associated with lower total doses of radiation and increased functional outcomes. However, preoperative radiation therapy carries with it a higher risk of postoperative wound healing issues.[42] Some clinicians have advocated for a postoperative radiation boost in patients treated with radiation therapy preoperatively with positive surgical margins. This is controversial, however, and a recent study demonstrated no reduction in local recurrence with employment of this strategy.[44]

CHEMOTHERAPY

Chemotherapy is generally reserved for patients with high-grade, large, deep soft tissue sarcomas and remains controversial. Most chemotherapy regimens for treatment of soft tissue sarcomas are based on doxorubicin. Any benefit of chemotherapy must be weighed against its potential toxicities. Several studies have suggested a modest benefit to chemotherapy, including a Cochrane review analyzing more than 1600 subjects from 14 randomized control trials that showed chemotherapy prolongs overall recurrence-free survival.[39,45–47] There are ongoing efforts to further characterize soft tissue sarcomas on a molecular level with the goal of providing improved understanding of the pathogenesis of these cancers, discovering potential therapeutic targets, and allowing for evaluation of response to different therapies.[48]

Table 2		
Classification of surgical margins described by Enneking		
Classification	**Definition**	**Notes**
Intralesional	Margins within mass	Incisional biopsy
Marginal	Margins at immediate border of tumor	Excisional biopsy
Wide	Margins include cuff of normal tissue beyond boundary of tumor	Most resections for soft tissue sarcomas
Radical	Margins include entire compartment in which tumor is confined	Rarely used

SUMMARY

Soft tissue sarcomas are rare but given their potential for patient morbidity and mortality the diagnosis should be on the differential for any soft tissue mass. Soft tissue sarcomas generally present with nonspecific clinical and radiographic features. The absence of pain or constitutional symptoms is not helpful in differentiating benign from malignant soft tissue masses. Masses deep to the fascia and those larger than 5 cm are more likely to represent soft tissue sarcomas; however, approximately one-third of soft tissue sarcomas will present as superficial masses. Any patient with an indeterminate soft tissue mass or a patient who undergoes unplanned resection of a soft tissue sarcoma should be referred in a timely manner to a tumor specialty center with a multidisciplinary sarcoma team. Biopsies for masses suspicious for soft tissue sarcoma should be performed at a specialty center.

REFERENCES

1. Wiklund T, Huuhtanen R, Blomqvist C, et al. The importance of a multidisciplinary group in the treatment of soft tissue sarcomas. Eur J Cancer 1996; 32A(2):269–73.

2. Gustafson P, Dreinhofer KE, Rydholm A. Soft tissue sarcoma should be treated at a tumor center. A comparison of quality of surgery in 375 patients. Acta Orthop Scand 1994;65(1):47–50.

3. Siegel R, Ward E, Brawley O, et al. Cancer statistics, 2011. CA Cancer J Clin 2011;61(4):212–36.

4. Esther R. Soft-tissue sarcomas. In: Biermann J, editor. Orthopaedic Knowledge update. Chicago: American Academy of Orthopaedic Surgeons; 2013. p. 295–306.

5. Bauer HC, Trovik CS, Alvegard TA, et al. Monitoring referral and treatment in soft tissue sarcoma: study based on 1,851 patients from the Scandinavian Sarcoma Group Register. Acta Orthop Scand 2001; 72(2):150–9.

6. Damron TA, Beauchamp CP, Rougraff BT, et al. Soft-tissue lumps and bumps. Instr Course Lect 2004;53: 625–37.

7. Riad S, Biau D, Holt GE, et al. The clinical and functional outcome for patients with radiation-induced soft tissue sarcoma. Cancer 2012;118(10):2682–92.

8. Li-Fraumeni Syndrome - GeneReviews® - NCBI Bookshelf. 2014. Available at: http://www.ncbi.nlm. nih.gov/books/NBK1116. Accessed December 6, 2014.

9. Pike J, Clarkson PW, Marsi BA. Soft tissue sarcomas of the extremities; How to stay out of trouble. BC Medical Journal 2008;50(6):310–7.

10. Ferguson PC, Griffin AM, O'Sullivan B, et al. Bone invasion in extremity soft-tissue sarcoma: impact on disease outcomes. Cancer 2006;106(12):2692–700.

11. Doyle AJ, Miller MV, French JG. Ultrasound of soft-tissue masses: pitfalls in interpretation. Australas Radiol 2000;44(3):275–80.

12. Papp DF, Khanna AJ, McCarthy EF, et al. Magnetic resonance imaging of soft-tissue tumors: determinate and indeterminate lesions. J Bone Joint Surg Am 2007;89(Suppl 3):103–15.

13. Ward WG Sr, Rougraff B, Quinn R, et al. Tumors masquerading as hematomas. Clin Orthop Relat Res 2007;465:232–40.

14. Huang AJ, Kattapuram SV. Musculoskeletal neoplasms: biopsy and intervention. Radiol Clin North Am 2011;49(6):1287–305, vii.

15. Mankin HJ, Mankin CJ, Simon MA. The hazards of the biopsy, revisited. Members of the Musculoskeletal Tumor Society. J Bone Joint Surg Am 1996; 78(5):656–63.

16. Verheijen P, Witjes H, van Gorp J, et al. Current pathology work-up of extremity soft tissue sarcomas, evaluation of the validity of different techniques. Eur J Surg Oncol 2010;36(1):95–9.

17. Kasraeian S, Allison DC, Ahlmann ER, et al. A comparison of fine-needle aspiration, core biopsy, and surgical biopsy in the diagnosis of extremity soft tissue masses. Clin Orthop Relat Res 2010;468(11): 2992–3002.

18. Heslin MJ, Lewis JJ, Woodruff JM, et al. Core needle biopsy for diagnosis of extremity soft tissue sarcoma. Ann Surg Oncol 1997;4(5):425–31.

19. Ray-Coquard I, Ranchere-Vince D, Thiesse P, et al. Evaluation of core needle biopsy as a substitute to open biopsy in the diagnosis of soft-tissue masses. Eur J Cancer 2003;39(14):2021–5.

20. Narvani AA, Tsiridis E, Saifuddin A, et al. Does image guidance improve accuracy of core needle biopsy in diagnosis of soft tissue tumours? Acta Orthop Belg 2009;75(2):239–44.

21. Pohlig F, Kirchhoff C, Lenze U, et al. Percutaneous core needle biopsy versus open biopsy in diagnostics of bone and soft tissue sarcoma: a retrospective study. Eur J Med Res 2012;17:29.

22. Mayerson JL, Scharschmidt TJ, Lewis VO, et al. Diagnosis and Management of Soft-tissue Masses. J Am Acad Orthop Surg 2014;22(11):742–50.

23. Giuliano AE, Eilber FR. The rationale for planned reoperation after unplanned total excision of soft-tissue sarcomas. J Clin Oncol 1985;3(10):1344–8.

24. Qureshi YA, Huddy JR, Miller JD, et al. Unplanned excision of soft tissue sarcoma results in increased rates of local recurrence despite full further oncological treatment. Ann Surg Oncol 2012;19(3):871–7.

25. Lewis JJ, Leung D, Espat J, et al. Effect of reresection in extremity soft tissue sarcoma. Ann Surg 2000; 231(5):655–63.

26. Noria S, Davis A, Kandel R, et al. Residual disease following unplanned excision of soft-tissue sarcoma of an extremity. J Bone Joint Surg Am 1996;78(5):650–5.

27. Fiore M, Casali PG, Miceli R, et al. Prognostic effect of re-excision in adult soft tissue sarcoma of the extremity. Ann Surg Oncol 2006;13(1):110–7.

28. Zagars GK, Ballo MT, Pisters PW, et al. Surgical margins and reresection in the management of patients with soft tissue sarcoma using conservative surgery and radiation therapy. Cancer 2003;97(10):2544–53.

29. Manoso MW, Frassica DA, Deune EG, et al. Outcomes of re-excision after unplanned excisions of soft-tissue sarcomas. J Surg Oncol 2005;91(3):153–8.

30. Coindre JM, Terrier P, Bui NB, et al. Prognostic factors in adult patients with locally controlled soft tissue sarcoma. A study of 546 patients from the French Federation of Cancer Centers Sarcoma Group. J Clin Oncol 1996;14(3):869–77.

31. Pisters PW, Leung DH, Woodruff J, et al. Analysis of prognostic factors in 1,041 patients with localized soft tissue sarcomas of the extremities. J Clin Oncol 1996;14(5):1679–89.

32. Maretty-Nielsen K, Aggerholm-Pedersen N, Keller J, et al. Relative mortality in soft tissue sarcoma patients: a Danish population-based cohort study. BMC Cancer 2014;14:682.

33. Abatzoglou S, Turcotte RE, Adoubali A, et al. Local recurrence after initial multidisciplinary management of soft tissue sarcoma: is there a way out? Clin Orthop Relat Res 2010;468(11):3012–8.

34. Gibbs CP, Peabody TD, Mundt AJ, et al. Oncological outcomes of operative treatment of subcutaneous soft-tissue sarcomas of the extremities. J Bone Joint Surg Am 1997;79(6):888–97.

35. Peabody TD, Monson D, Montag A, et al. A comparison of the prognoses for deep and subcutaneous sarcomas of the extremities. J Bone Joint Surg Am 1994;76(8):1167–73.

36. Potter BK, Adams SC, Qadir R, et al. Fungating soft-tissue sarcomas. Treatment implications and prognostic importance of malignant ulceration. J Bone Joint Surg Am 2009;91(3):567–74.

37. Biau DJ, Ferguson PC, Turcotte RE, et al. Adverse effect of older age on the recurrence of soft tissue sarcoma of the extremities and trunk. J Clin Oncol 2011;29(30):4029–35.

38. Binitie O, Tejiram S, Conway S, et al. Adult soft tissue sarcoma local recurrence after adjuvant treatment without resection of core needle biopsy tract. Clin Orthop Relat Res 2013;471(3):891–8.

39. Rosenberg SA, Tepper J, Glatstein E, et al. The treatment of soft-tissue sarcomas of the extremities: prospective randomized evaluations of (1) limb-sparing surgery plus radiation therapy compared with amputation and (2) the role of adjuvant chemotherapy. Ann Surg 1982;196(3):305–15.

40. Clarkson PW, Griffin AM, Catton CN, et al. Epineural dissection is a safe technique that facilitates limb salvage surgery. Clin Orthop Relat Res 2005;438:92–6.

41. Rosenberg LA, Esther RJ, Erfanian K, et al. Wound complications in preoperatively irradiated soft-tissue sarcomas of the extremities. Int J Radiat Oncol Biol Phys 2013;85(2):432–7.

42. O'Sullivan B, Davis AM, Turcotte R, et al. Preoperative versus postoperative radiotherapy in soft-tissue sarcoma of the limbs: a randomised trial. Lancet 2002;359(9325):2235–41.

43. Sawamura C, Springfield DS, Marcus KJ, et al. Factors predicting local recurrence, metastasis, and survival in pediatric soft tissue sarcoma in extremities. Clin Orthop Relat Res 2010;468(11):3019–27.

44. Pan E, Goldberg SI, Chen YL, et al. Role of postoperative radiation boost for soft tissue sarcomas with positive margins following pre-operative radiation and surgery. J Surg Oncol 2014;110(7):817–22.

45. Rosenberg SA, Tepper J, Glatstein E, et al. Prospective randomized evaluation of adjuvant chemotherapy in adults with soft tissue sarcomas of the extremities. Cancer 1983;52(3):424–34.

46. Sarcoma Meta-analysis Collaboration (SMAC). Adjuvant chemotherapy for localised resectable soft tissue sarcoma in adults. Cochrane Database Syst Rev 2000;(4):CD001419.

47. Pervaiz N, Colterjohn N, Farrokhyar F, et al. A systematic meta-analysis of randomized controlled trials of adjuvant chemotherapy for localized resectable soft-tissue sarcoma. Cancer 2008;113(3):573–81.

48. Neuville A, Chibon F, Coindre JM. Grading of soft tissue sarcomas: from histological to molecular assessment. Pathology 2014;46(2):113–20.

Index

Note: Page numbers of article titles are in **boldface** type.

A

Acetaminophen
  after hand surgery, 403
Acromioclavicular joint reconstruction
  acellular human dermal allograft for, 384–385
Analgesia/analgesics
  hand surgery–related, 400–404
Anesthesia/anesthetics
  hand surgery–related, 400–402
Arthroplasty. *See specific types, e.g.,* Total hip
  arthroplasty (THA)

B

Biologic glenoid resurfacing
  acellular human dermal allograft for, 384
Blood loss
  in bilateral TKA
    patient-specific instrumentation in reducing,
    343–350. *See also* Total knee arthroplasty
    (TKA), bilateral, reducing blood loss in,
    patient-specific instrumentation in

C

Chemotherapy
  for soft tissue masses, 426
Computed tomography (CT)
  PET with
    in sarcoma, **409–415**. *See also* Sarcoma(s),
    PET/CT imaging in
Continuous peripheral nerve blockade (CPNB)
  after hand surgery, 404
CPNB. *See* Continuous peripheral nerve blockade
  (CPNB)
CT. *See* Computed tomography (CT)

D

Dermal allograft
  acellular human
    for elbow surgery, **377–380, 385–387**
      future applications in, 387
      introduction, 377–378
      orthopedic applications, **377–380, 385–387**
        distal biceps tendon repair, 385–387
      options for, 378–380
      safety of, 380
    for shoulder surgery, **377–385**
      introduction, 377–378

      orthopedic applications, **377–385**
        acromioclavicular joint reconstruction,
        384–385
        biologic glenoid resurfacing, 384
        pectoralis major tendon repair, 384
        rotator cuff tears, 380–384
    basics of, 378–380
Distal biceps tendon repair
  acellular human dermal allograft for, 387

E

Elbow surgery
  acellular human dermal allograft for, **377–380,
  385–387**. *See also* Dermal allograft, acellular
  human, for elbow surgery
Extended local blocks
  after hand surgery, 405
Extended peripheral nerve blocks
  after hand surgery, 405–406

F

Femoral bone loss
  causes of, 329
  classifications of, 330
  in revision THA, **329–342**
    management of, **329–342**
      femoral component removal in, 332–336
      options and outcomes for specific bone
        defects, 336–340
        type I defects, 336–337
        type II defects, 337
        type IIIA defects, 337
        type IIIB defects, 337–338
        type IV defects, 338–340
      radiographic and clinical patient evaluation
        in, 330–332
      surgical approach in, 332
Fracture(s). *See also specific types, e.g.,* Tibial
  plateau fractures
  tibial plateau
    definitive fixation of, **363–375**. *See also* Tibial
    plateau fractures

G

General anesthesia
  for hand surgery, 400
Glenoid bone loss
  in anatomic shoulder arthroplasty, **389–397**

Orthop Clin N Am 46 (2015) 429–431
http://dx.doi.org/10.1016/S0030-5898(15)00073-5
0030-5898/15/$ – see front matter © 2015 Elsevier Inc. All rights reserved.

orthopedic.theclinics.com

Glenoid (*continued*)
    B2 glenoid
        surgical treatment of, 389–391
            anterior reaming, 393
            asymmetric reaming and glenoid
                resurfacing, 390
            augmented polyethylene glenoid,
                390–391
            bone grafting, 390
            bone preparation assessment and
                tamping, 394
            drilling peripheral peg holes, 394–395
            posterior preparation, 393–394
            preoperative planning, 392–393
            ream and run, 390
            reverse arthroplasty, 391
            sizer pin guide placement and sizing,
                392–393
            technique, 392
            trialing/final implant, 395–396
    C glenoids
        surgical treatment of, 391–396
            indications for, 391–392
    discussion, 396
    introduction, 389

H

Hand surgery
    pain management strategies in, **399–408**
        future directions in, 404–406
            CPNB, 404
            extended local blocks, 405
            extended peripheral nerve blocks, 405–406
        intraoperative analgesia, 400–402
            general anesthesia, 400
            intravenous regional anesthesia, 401
            peripheral regional blocks, 400–401
            wide-awake surgery–related, 401–402
        introduction, 399–400
        postoperative analgesia, 402–404
            home analgesia, 402–403
            opioids, 403–404
            postanesthesia care unit, 402
Highly cross-linked polyethylene (HXLPE)
    in THA, **321–327**
        described, 323–324
        introduction, 321–323
    in TKA, **321–327**
        described, 324–325
        introduction, 321–323
    vitamin E stabilized, 325
HXLPE. *See* Highly cross-linked polyethylene
    (HXLPE)

I

Intravenous regional anesthesia
    for hand surgery, 401

K

Ketorolac
    after hand surgery, 403

L

Latissimus dorsi tendon transfers
    acellular human dermal allograft for
        in rotator cuff tear management, 383–384

M

Massachusetts General Hospital
    experience with risk assessment and prediction
        tools after THA and TKA, 360–361

N

Nerve blocks
    hand surgery–related, 400–401, 405–406
Nonsteroidal antiinflammatory drugs (NSAIDs)
    after hand surgery, 403

O

Opioid(s)
    after hand surgery, 403–404

P

Pain
    hand surgery–related
        management of, **399–408**. *See also* Hand
            surgery, pain management strategies in
Pectoralis major tendon repair
    acellular human dermal allograft for, 384
Peripheral nerve blocks
    extended
        after hand surgery, 405–406
Peripheral regional blocks
    for hand surgery, 400–401
PET. *See* Positron emission tomography (PET)
Positron emission tomography (PET)
    background of, 409
    principle of, 409–410
    in sarcoma, **409–415**. *See also* Sarcoma(s),
        PET/CT imaging in
Positron emission tomography (PET)/computed
    tomography (CT)
    in sarcoma, **409–415**. *See also* Sarcoma(s),
        PET/CT imaging in
Prediction tools
    in THA and TKA outcomes, **351–362**
        demand for, 353
        for discharge to extended care facilities,
            353–354
        introduction, 351–353
        length of stay–related, 357

Massachusetts General Hospital experience
with, 360–361
for patient functional outcomes, 358–360
for postoperative complications, 354–357
for postoperative ICU monitoring, 357
for successful treatment of prosthetic joint
infections, 358
Prosthetic joint infections
after THA or TKA
management of
prediction tools in, 358

R

Radiation therapy
for soft tissue masses, 425–426
Rotator cuff tears
acellular human dermal allograft for, 380–384
latissimus dorsi tendon transfers, 383–384
superior capsular reconstruction, 382–383

S

Sarcoma(s)
PET/CT imaging in
applications, 410–413
in biopsy guidance, 410–411
in detection and grading, 410
in prognostication, 413
in staging, 411–412
in therapeutic monitoring, 412–413
PET imaging in, **409–415**
Shoulder surgery
acellular human dermal allograft for, **377–385**. See
also Dermal allograft, acellular human, for
shoulder surgery
Soft tissue masses
for general orthopedic surgeon, **417–428**
biopsy, 419, 422
chemotherapy, 426
clinical presentation, 417–418, 420–421
evaluation, 417–418
introduction, 417
prognosis, 423–424
radiation therapy, 425–426
radiographic findings, 418–421
surgical management, 424–425
unplanned resections, 422–423
Superior capsular reconstruction
acellular human dermal allograft for
in rotator cuff tear management, 382–383

T

THA. See Total hip arthroplasty (THA)
Thromboembolism
blood loss reduction measures in bilateral TKA
and, 347

Tibial plateau fractures
definitive fixation of, **363–375**
after soft tissue resolution, 364–365
case-based strategies and techniques,
365–373
complex fractures, 370–373
fracture-dislocations, 367–369
simple split fractures, 365–367
split-depression fractures, 367
considerations before, 364
introduction, 363
TKA. See Total knee arthroplasty (TKA)
Total hip arthroplasty (THA)
background of, 329
demand for, 351
HXLPE in, **321–327**. See also Highly cross-linked
polyethylene (HXLPE), in THA
outcomes of
risk assessment tools in predicting, **351–362**.
See also Prediction tools, in THA and TKA
outcomes
revision
femoral bone loss in
management of, **329–342**. See also Femoral
bone loss, in revision THA
Total knee arthroplasty (TKA)
bilateral
reducing blood loss in
patient-specific instrumentation in,
343–350
complications of, 345–347
discussion, 347–349
Introduction, 343–344
limitations of, 347, 349
methods, 344–345
outcomes of, 345
study aims, 344
surgical time in, 347
demand for, 351
HXLPE in, **321–327**. See also Highly cross-linked
polyethylene (HXLPE), in TKA
outcomes of
risk assessment tools in predicting, **351–362**.
See also Prediction tools, in THA and TKA
outcomes
Total shoulder arthroplasty (TSA)
glenoid bone loss in, **389–397**. See also Glenoid
bone loss, in anatomic shoulder arthroplasty
TSA. See Total shoulder arthroplasty (TSA)

V

Vitamin E stabilized HXLPE, 325

W

Wide-awake hand surgery
pain management strategies for, 401–402

Moving?

Make sure your subscription moves with you!

To notify us of your new address, find your **Clinics Account Number** (located on your mailing label above your name), and contact customer service at:

Email: journalscustomerservice-usa@elsevier.com

800-654-2452 (subscribers in the U.S. & Canada)
314-447-8871 (subscribers outside of the U.S. & Canada)

Fax number: 314-447-8029

Elsevier Health Sciences Division
Subscription Customer Service
3251 Riverport Lane
Maryland Heights, MO 63043

*To ensure uninterrupted delivery of your subscription, please notify us at least 4 weeks in advance of move.

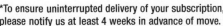

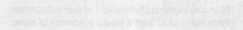

Printed and bound by CPI Group (UK) Ltd, Croydon, CR0 4YY

03/10/2024

01040375-0010